Simple Keto Diet Cookbook:

Easy Keto Recipes for Pizza,

Sandwiches, Pates,

Desserts and Snacks.

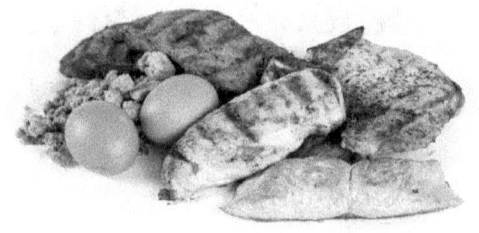

Dana Patton

Contents

INTRODUCTION

If you're looking to lose weight, then consider restricting your carbohydrate intake. By using techniques such as the Ketogenic diet, you can change your lifestyle completely. It is often used as a healthy nutrition plan for many athletics, especially endurance athletes.

You don't have to give up your favorite pizza and burgers in which carbohydrates predominate. You can just replace some ingredients and then pamper yourself with your favorite dishes because the number of carbohydrates in them will be consistent with the Ketogenic diet requirements.

Moreover, a person cannot exclude carbohydrates completely from food, as this can lead to a serious disruption of the digestive system. Also, fiber is necessary for normal digestion.

This book will help to complement your Keto diet with familiar dishes.

Ketogenic Diet is a Change in Lifestyle

Ketones for Energy

Normally, the food we eat is processed in the gut, then absorbed into the bloodstream. Once there, the body absorbs as many of the nutrients as possible. Those nutrients flow around the bloodstream where the liver changes them into glucose. It is glucose that uses for energy. However, when we produce too much glucose, such as when we don't burn it off, our body stores it away as fat. This is what leads to an increase in weight. A major source of too much sugar in the bloodstream is caused by excessive intake of carbohydrates, especially starchy ones.

The Keto diet involves eating healthy high-fat foods. Also included are medium amounts of protein and low carb meals. This stops the body from producing excess glucose. By cutting down on sugary carbs, it leads to insufficient glucose in the bloodstream. To provide the necessary energy our body still needs, we use the fatty acids that are stored away. The liver turns those fatty acids into ketones, the new energy source that has replaced glucose. This is the first stage of ketosis or lipolysis.

Health specialists worked on developing this diet to tackle severe epileptic cases that are difficult-to-control, in children. It is the ketone bodies in the bloodstream that competently block epileptic seizures.

Nowadays, this food system is being promoted to fight to be overweight and as a diet.

Types of Keto Diets

✓ SKD is the acronym for the Standard Ketogenic Diet which contains 75% of fat, 20% of protein, and 5% carbs. SKD is usually the first that nutritionists consider.

✓ Cyclic Ketogenic Diet Plan: Also known as CKD. Periodic repetition of carb administration. For example, five ketogenic days, and two high carb days.

✓ Targeted Ketogenic Diet: TKD is the kind of planned diet for physical training. It includes carbohydrates and higher-protein into the Keto diet. In practice, it is the same Keto diet. The difference is that it includes a higher amount of protein source into the meal. The percentage count is 60% fat, 35% protein, and 5% carbohydrates

Benefits of the Standard Ketogenic Diet (SKD)

Initially, the stored fat cells shrink as they lose the water they are stored within. This is the first phase of losing weight. Now that the fat cells are smaller, they can enter the bloodstream and go to the liver. The body's chemistry is changing, and all for the better. Why?

✓ Fat ketones are a more efficient energy source than glucose energy.

✓ For patients with Diabetes Type II, the zero sugars in the bloodstream allow them to control their condition better. This is because ketones also assist with balancing natural insulin production.

✓ For patients who suffer epilepsy, it is believed that the ketones in the bloodstream have an anticonvulsant effect.

✓ The body can only make so much glucose energy, so needs to constant refuel with more carbs to make more energy. Ketone energy is a constant supply, leading you to feel energetic for longer.

✓ Lower blood sugars lead to lower cholesterol levels, which in turn lowers blood pressure. Ketones help to increase healthy cholesterol, HDL, and decrease the unhealthy cholesterol, LDL. This reduces the chances of heart disease.

✓ Carbs have long been associated with poor skin conditions, such as acne. By reducing carbs in your diet, your skin condition should improve.

✓ Ketone energy is better for the brain. Not only improving concentration skills but also decreasing the chances of neurological diseases, such as Alzheimer's.

Other Keto diets are TKD and CKD though they are more specialist for athletes and bodybuilders.

Ketosis Good or Bad?

Ketosis is a natural adaptive metabolic condition. Our ancestors would have entered ketosis when between hunting sessions, or when food was scarce. Fasting is another way for the body to stop producing glucose for energy and enter ketosis. For those who choose to enter ketosis as part of their diet, then you need to eat less than 50 grams of carbs per day. After 3-4 days, your body will no longer produce glucose and ketosis will begin.

Entering a state of ketosis is not dangerous. It should not be confused with Diabetic Ketoacidosis. That is a medical condition that can be harmful to people with diabetes. The type of ketosis we are discussing here is nutritional ketosis. There are a few side effects though, and they can affect people in different ways. Initially, you may experience any of the following, but it's unlikely you will suffer them all:

- Decreased appetite.
- Bad breath and dry mouth.
- Fatigue and cloudy brain.

- Increased urination.
- Dizziness.
- Low blood sugars.
- Food cravings.
- Constipation.
- Unable to sleep.

Don't worry the symptoms are short-lived. They are only noticeable as your body enters the first metabolic changes. They are symptoms that you can manage, by:

- Drinking plenty of water.
- Slightly increasing your salt intake for a few days.
- Including plenty of healthy fats in your dietary intake.

Once ketosis kicks in, it means that your body is now using fat for energy and not glucose.

Transition to and Exit from the Keto Diet

Transition Process

It takes the human body close to two weeks to adapt to the Keto diet.

- ✓ Glucose Consumption: this stage occurs after 12 hours of a regular meal. The body burns all the glucose it already had from the last meal.

- ✓ Glycogen Consumption: this is when the body has exhausted its glucose supply. With the shortage of sugars now in the bloodline, the liver will use any glycogen found in muscles. It can take up to two days for the body to utilize its glycogen completely.

- ✓ Fat and Protein Consumption: a stage that begins when the body system has absorbed all the carbohydrate energy sources in the body. This moment is usually the hardest for the patient who is undergoing the diet. What the liver will do at this stage, is to start transforming stored fatty acids into the needed energy source. It also locates proteins in the muscles and other areas of the body, turning these amino components into energy.

✓ Ketosis (Fat Consumption): it is on the seventh day of this strict meal plan that the body completely adjusts to the new source of energy. At this stage, human anatomy has learned that there are no carbohydrates in the body, and so ketosis begins. The body slows down its intake of food protein, and relies primarily on fat.

Exit Process

To get out of the Keto diet plan, you need to gradually increase the carb content in the diet by 30 grams per day.

Who the Diet is Unsafe for?

Before going for a Keto diet plan, discuss it first with your nutritionist. Pregnant women cannot and should not follow a Keto diet plan.

Other people who cannot follow the program, are individuals suffering issues in the stomach-intestinal tract, kidney, liver, and those with thyroid gland issues.

What useful and what to avoid on the Keto diet

The different types of food available on the ketogenic diet plan, are delicious and full of variety. Your meals will not be boring. Your new diet will contain High fat, Medium protein and Low carbs.

You Can Eat
Meat

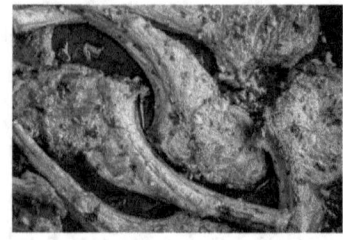

- Beef
- Lamb
- Goat Meat
- Venison
- Grass-fed Pork
- Domestic bird
- Liver
- Other meat by-products (if you eat them)

Avoid sausages and meat covered with breadcrumbs; meat that comes with a sweet or starchy sauce.

Fish and Seafood

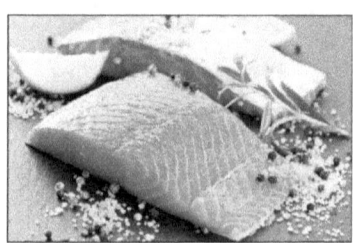

Most seafood is filled with omega-3 fatty acids, which have a significant impact on your overall health, especially on your cardiovascular system. They reduce the risk of heart disease and stroke, help lower triglyceride levels and blood pressure and increase your good cholesterol.

- Crab
- Lobster
- Oysters
- Salmon
- Shrimp

The only exceptions are some types of mollusks (for example, mussels). So, you need to be more careful with them and eat in small portions.

Eggs

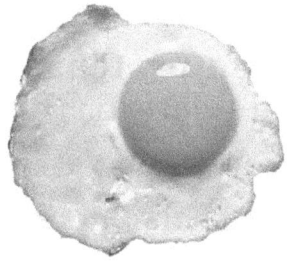

Healthy Fats

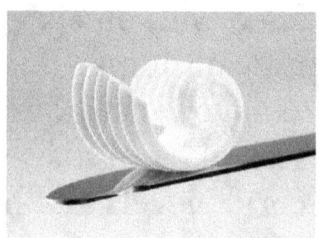

Saturated

- lard,
- fat,
- chicken fat,
- duck fat,
- goose fat,
- clarified butter / ghee oil,
- butter,
- coconut oil

Monounsaturated
- avocado,
- macadamia and olive oil

Omega-3 polyunsaturated fats, especially from animal sources (fatty fish and seafood)

Light Starchy Vegetables

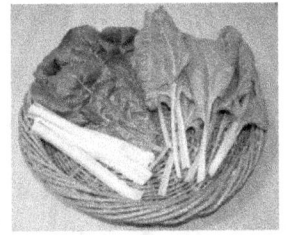

Leafy greens

- Swiss chard,
- bok choy,
- spinach,
- lettuce,
- chard,
- onion,
- endive,
- radicchio,
- etc.

- Broccoli,
- cauliflower,
- kohlrabi,
- radishes

- Celery stalk,
- asparagus,
- cucumber,
- zucchini,
- bamboo shoots

Fruits

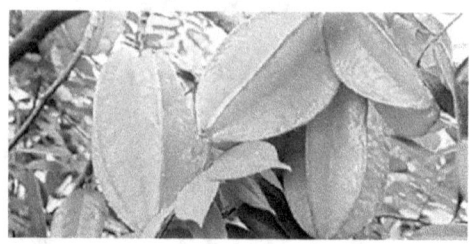

Because of fruits contain natural sugar (fructose), you should carefully monitor the amount of low-carbohydrate fruit you consume each day.

- Avocado
- Rhubarb
- Carambola

Beverages and Spices

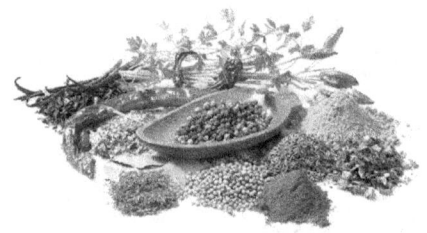

- Water,
- coffee (black, with cream or coconut milk),
- tea (black, herbal)

Use almond flour, coconut flour, pork rings or almond breadcrumbs to replace breadcrumbs

- Mayonnaise,
- mustard,
- pesto,
- bone broth,
- pickled cucumbers,
- fermented foods (kimchi, kombucha, and sauerkraut)

All spices and herbs,

Whey protein (beware of artificial sweeteners, hormones and soy lecithin), egg yolk and gelatin (without hormones)

You Can Eat from Time to Time

Vegetables, Mushrooms and Fruits

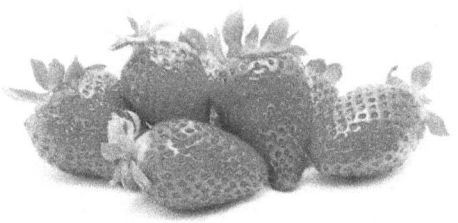

- Cabbage,
- red cabbage,

- Brussels sprouts,
- fennel,
- turnips
- Eggplants,
- tomatoes,
- peppers

Some root vegetables (parsley root);
- green onions,
- leeks,
- garlic,
- mushrooms,
- pumpkin

Sea vegetables (nori, kombu);
- okra,
- bean sprouts,
- sugar snap peas,
- wax beans,
- artichoke,
- water chestnuts

Berries
- blackberries,
- blueberries,
- strawberries,
- raspberries,
- cranberries,
- etc.

- Coconut,
- Olives

Full-fat Dairy Products

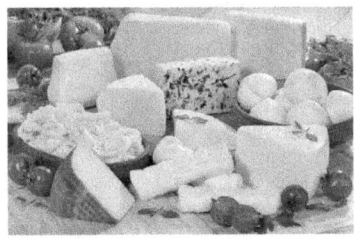

- Blue cheese
- Brie
- Cheddar cheese
- Colby Jack Cheese
- Cottage cheese
- Cream cheese
- Cheese Feta
- Goat cheese
- Gouda
- Full Fat Plain Yogurt
- Full Fat Greek Yogurt
- Heavy whipping cream
- Mozzarella cheese
- Parmesan cheese
- Provolone cheese
- Ricotta
- Sour cream
- Cream

- Swiss cheese

Nuts and Seeds

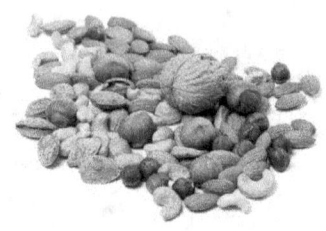

- Macadamia Nuts (very few carbohydrates)
- Pecans,
- almonds,
- walnuts,
- hazelnuts,
- pine nuts,
- flaxseed,
- pumpkin seeds,
- sesame seeds,
- sunflower seeds
- Brazil nuts (beware of very high amounts of selenium - do not eat them too much!)

Cooking Ingredients

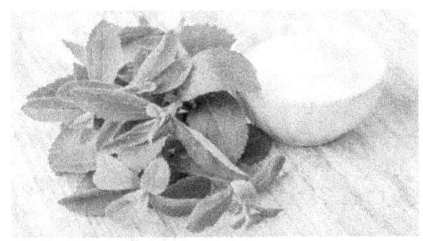

Healthy sweeteners

- stevia,
- erythritol,
- etc.

Thickeners:

- purple powder,
- xanthan gum

Tomato products without sugar
- mashed potatoes,
- trade winds,
- ketchup

- Cocoa,
- dark chocolate (with a cocoa content of more than 70%, but better than 90% and beware of soy lecithin),
- cocoa powder
-

You can't eat

All grains, even in the form of flour (wheat, rye, oats, corn, barley, millet, bulgur, sorghum, rice, amaranth, buckwheat, sprouted grains), quinoa and white potatoes. This includes all grain products (pasta, bread, pizza, cookies, crackers, etc.)

Sugar and sweets (table sugar, corn syrup, agave syrup, ice cream, cakes, sweet puddings and sweet non-alcoholic beverages). Beware of sugar-free chewing gums - some of them contain carbohydrates.

Tropical fruits (pineapple, mango, banana, papaya, etc.) and some fruits that are high in carbohydrates (mandarin, grapes, etc.)

Also avoid fruit juices (yes, even 100% fresh juices!) and dried fruits - dates, raisins, etc. (if they are in large quantities).

Alcoholic, sweet drinks (beer, sweet wine, cocktails, etc.).

Always remember, you do not need to worry about your fat intake on the Keto diet. Just ensure you are not eating unhealthy "unsaturated" fats. Use Olive oil to cook with and not vegetable oil. When buying foods, check the labels for the sugar content, and check that it uses "saturated" fats. While you may seem to think it odd that "saturated" fats are included in this diet, they have been unfairly maligned over the last few decades. "Saturated" fats are essential for a healthy immune system.

For those who not athletically minded, you still need to include simple exercise in your daily regime. A minimum of 20 minutes a day is good for your diet, also good for your heart and mind. Find pleasant walks; leave your desk at lunchtime; or go for a swim once a week. There are many ways to incorporate simple exercises into your life, without overexerting yourself.

Why Choose the Ketogenic Diet?

One of the main benefits and probably the reason you are embarking on a Ketonic diet is weight loss. The major reason for continued weight loss when on the Keto diet, is that you don't feel as hungry. This in turn reduces your appetite.

The type of energy that burning fat produces is more efficient than the energy produced by burning sugar. Compare it to buying a cheap battery that quickly runs out. Or, buy a more expensive one that not only lasts longer, but provides improved power. This improved energy source also helps our bodies to age slower.

If you have type two diabetes, then the Keto diet is a great way to reduce your blood sugar levels. This, in part, is due to the increase in insulin efficiency. A reduction in blood glucose levels can lead to less dependency on diabetic medication. A Keto diet will also help reduce the risk of you contracting type two diabetes.

A Keto diet can also help to lower blood pressure. A study published in 2007 shows that by eating fewer carbs, such as in the Keto diet, it can reduce both the systolic and diastolic pressure, of a blood pressure test.

Even Though the Keto diet is high in fats, albeit good fats, it helps reduce your cholesterol levels. Even better, the good cholesterol, HDL, in your bloodstream will increase. The ratio between good cholesterol and bad, LDL, should be around 3.5. The Keto diet will help you achieve this figure.

The Keto diet is high in healthy fats such as omega -3. Such fats help produce DHA, a fatty acid that makes up almost a third of brain matter. This increases positive mood swings and increases the ability to learn.

As you can see, there are plenty of benefits for your health, should you choose to follow the Keto diet. Don't be dissuaded by the fat component of the diet: fat has proven not to be the nemesis to good health. Gain a healthier lifestyle with the Keto diet and improve your health significantly.

Keto pizza

Most of the carbohydrates in pizza are in its dough. In this section, you will learn how to make a pizza dough with minimum carbohydrate content, and it will not spoil the taste of pizza at all. The recipe for making pizza keto crust is described in great detail with many photos. Shown below are recipes for your favorite pizzas that are suitable for Keto diets with calories, proteins, fats, and carbohydrates.

Cream-Cheese Keto Crust (for pizza)

Nutrients per 100 g:
- Total Carbs – 3.8 g
- Fat – 49.6 g
- Protein – 25.3 g
- Calories – 552.4

Ingredients:
- 100 g full-fat cream cheese
- 3 eggs
- 1/4 tsp salt

Directions:

1. Separate egg whites from yolks.

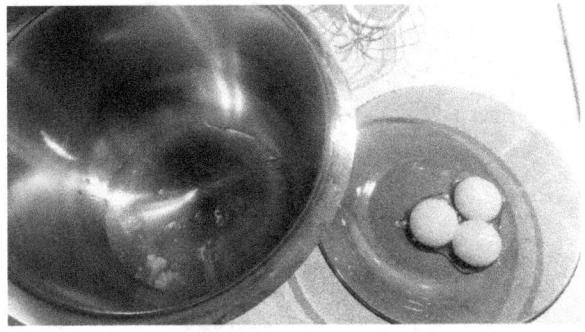

2. Preheat oven to 300°F

3. Beat egg whites with salt until dense foam.

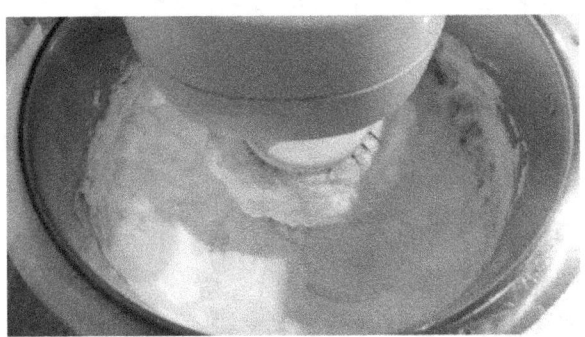

4. Mix yolks and cream cheese.

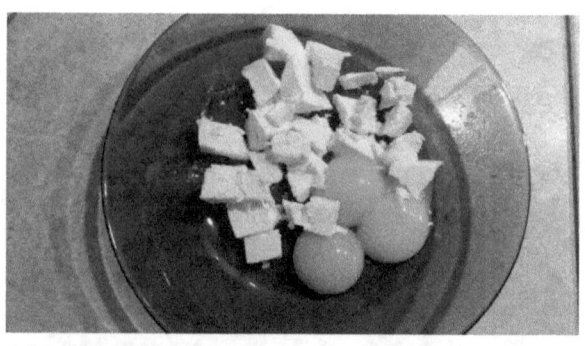

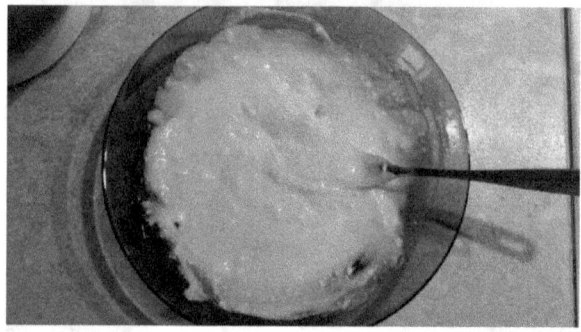

5. Combine the two mixtures with a spoon very neatly.

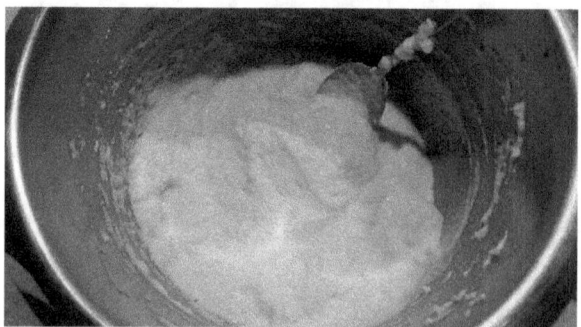

6. Cover the baking sheet with parchment paper.

7. Put the dough on the parchment paper and form a circle with a spoon.

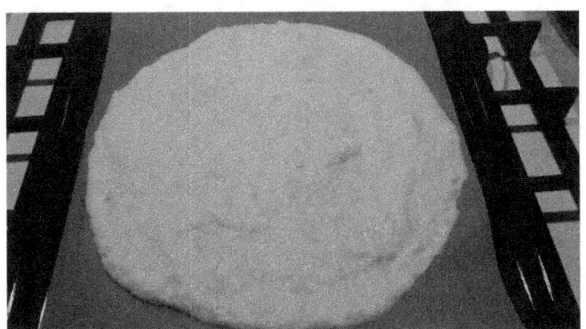

8. Bake for 25 minutes until crust is golden brown.

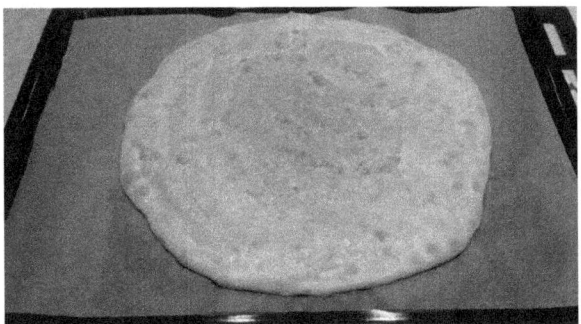

American Pizzas
St. Louis-Style Pizza

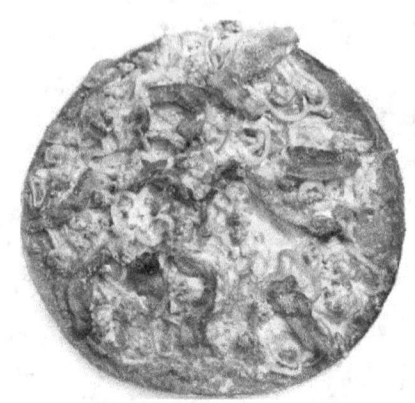

Nutrients per 100 g:
- Total Carbohydrates – 4.4 g
- Fat – 28.3 g
- Protein – 20.3 g
- Calories – 350.9

Ingredients:
- 1/3 cup pizza sauce
- 1/2 cup shredded white cheddar cheese
- 1/4 cup shredded smoked provolone
- 1/4 cup shredded Swiss cheese
- 1 teaspoon dried Italian or pizza seasoning

- 4 bacon strips
- 1/2 thinly sliced onion
- 1/2 thinly sliced seeded bell pepper

Directions:
1. Cook cream cheese keto crust as stated above.
2. Remove crust from the oven and increase oven temperature to 450°F.
3. Spread baked keto crust with pizza sauce.
4. Top with bacon strips, onion, and bell pepper.
5. Mix the cheeses and sprinkle with Italian herbs or pizza seasoning.
6. Bake until cheese is melted (from 5 to 10 minutes). Serve.

New-York style pizza

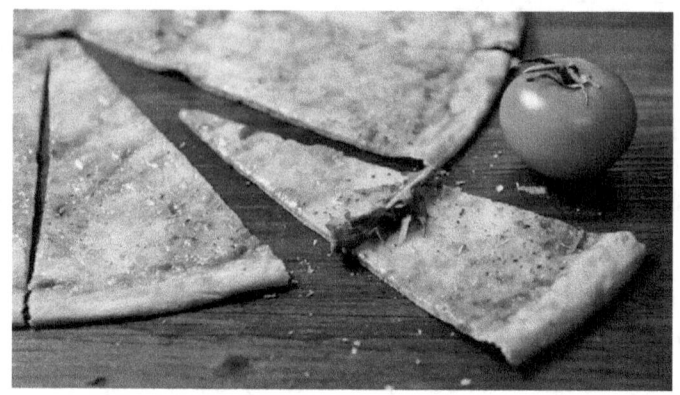

Nutrients per 100 g:
- Total Carbohydrates – 4.7 g
- Fat – 24.3 g
- Protein – 20 g
- Calories – 314.4

Ingredients:
- 1/2 cup pizza sauce
- 2 ¼ cup shredded mozzarella
- 1/2 cup grated parmesan cheese
- 2 garlic cloves, minced
- 1 teaspoon dried oregano
- 1 teaspoon red pepper flakes or optional

Directions:

1. Cook cream cheese keto crust as stated above.
2. Remove crust from the oven and increase oven temperature to 450°F.
2. Spread pizza sauce on baked keto crust.
3. Sprinkle with garlic, dried oregano, mozzarella and Parmesan cheese, and red pepper flakes.
4. Bake until cheese is melted. Slice and serve immediately.

New Haven-Style Clam Pizza

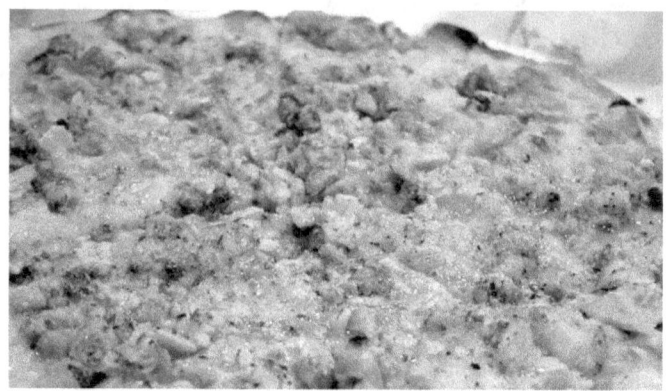

Nutrients per 100 g:
- Total Carbohydrates – 4.6 g
- Fat – 28 g
- Protein – 21.2 g
- Calories – 357.7

Ingredients:
- 1/2 cup grated Pecorino Romano
- 2 garlic cloves, minced
- 1/8 cup extra-virgin olive oil
- 12 littleneck clams, shucked, cooked
- 1 teaspoon dried oregano, crumbled

Directions:

1. Mix garlic and oil. Cover the mixture and chill.
2. Cook cream cheese keto crust as stated above.
3. While crust is cooking, let garlic oil come to room temperature.
4. Remove crust from the oven and increase oven temperature to 450°F.
5. Brush dough evenly with garlic oil. Arrange clams over garlic oil and sprinkle with oregano and Romano.
6. Bake about for 10 minutes until cheese is melted, slice and serve hot.

Greece-style Pizza

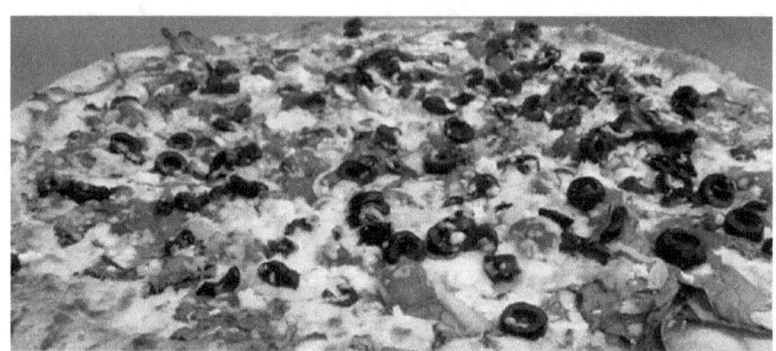

Nutrients per 100 g:
- Total Carbohydrates – 5.3 g
- Fat – 21.5 g
- Protein – 12.8 g
- Calories – 263.4

Ingredients:
- 2 teaspoons olive oil
- 1 cup shredded mozzarella
- 1 (6 ounces) bag prewashed baby spinach
- 3/4 cup pizza sauce
- 1 cup crumbled feta cheese
- 1/2 teaspoon ground pepper
- 1 (2 1/4-ounce) can black olives, sliced and drained
- 1 teaspoon dried oregano

Directions:
1. Cook spinach in an oiled nonstick skillet over medium-high heat for 3 minutes or until lightly wilted.
2. Cook cream cheese keto crust as stated above.
3. Remove crust from the oven and increase oven temperature to 450°F.
4. Spread baked keto crust with pizza sauce, dried oregano, and mozzarella.
5. Top with cooked spinach, feta cheese, pepper, and olives.
6. Bake until cheese is melted. Serve and enjoy!

Chicago style thin-crust Pizza

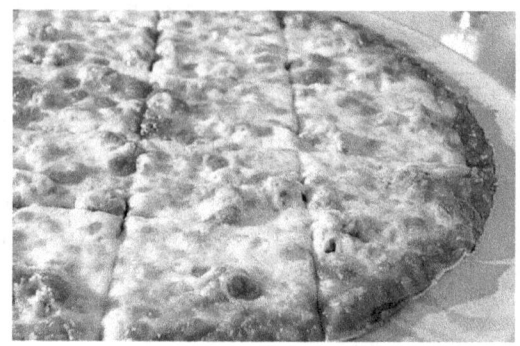

Nutrients per 100 g:
- Total Carbohydrates – 4.3 g
- Fat – 26.9 g
- Protein – 15.8 g
- Calories – 322.9

Ingredients:
- 4 oz. pepperoni
- 1 cup ground pork
- 2 jalapeños, sliced thinly
- 2 oz. sliced mushrooms
- 1 thinly sliced onion
- 1/2 teaspoon fennel seeds, crushed
- 3/4 cup pizza sauce
- 1/2 cup each of Smoked Provolone, Swiss and White Cheddar, grated and blended
- 1/8 cup extra-virgin olive oil

- 1 teaspoon dried oregano

Directions:
1. In a large nonstick skillet cook jalapeños, onion, and mushrooms with 2 teaspoons of oil for 7-10 minutes over medium-high heat. Remove to cool.
2. Roast the ground pork and add the oil, fennel, and salt and pepper (to taste).
3. Cook cream cheese keto crust as stated above.
4. Remove crust from the oven and increase oven temperature to 450°F.
5. Spread baked keto crust with pizza sauce, dried oregano, the pepperoni, and cheese.
6. Top with the ground pork, onion, jalapeños, and mushrooms.
7. Bake about 12 minutes or until cheese is melted. Cool for 10 minutes, and then slice and enjoy!

California-Style Barbecue Chicken Pizza

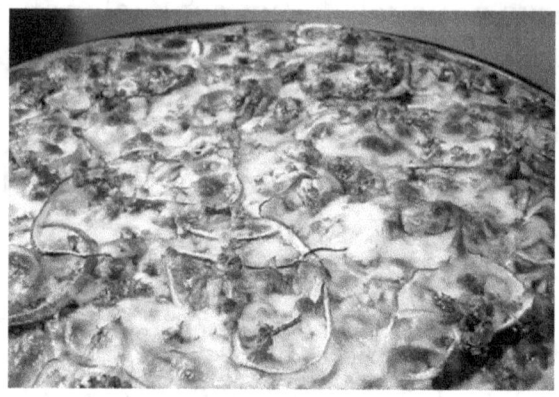

Nutrients per 100 g:
- Total Carbohydrates – 3.3 g
- Fat – 18.7 g
- Protein – 18.3 g
- Calories – 252.4

Ingredients:
- 8 ounces cooked chicken, chopped
- 1/3 cup prepared barbecue sauce, divided
- 1/2 cup shredded smoked Gouda cheese
- 3/4 cup shredded mozzarella cheese
- 1/2 small red onion, thinly sliced
- 2 tablespoons chopped fresh cilantro

Directions:

1. Toss the chicken with 2 tablespoons of barbecue sauce and set aside.
2. Cook cream cheese keto crust as stated above.
3. Remove crust from the oven and increase oven temperature to 450°F.
4. Spread baked keto crust with the remaining barbecue sauce and then scatter the chicken on top.
5. Top the pizza with the Gouda and mozzarella cheeses, and then with the onion.
6. Bake until cheese is melted. Sprinkle the cilantro before serving.

Grandma Pizza

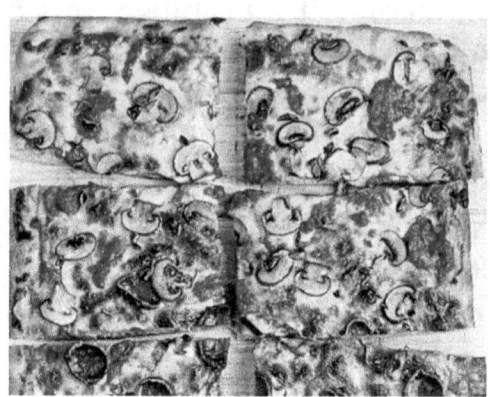

Nutrients per 100 g:
- Total Carbohydrates – 3.9 g
- Fat – 28.5 g
- Protein – 16.9 g
- Calories – 338.7

Ingredients:
- 2 tablespoons extra-virgin olive oil
- 2 ounces thinly sliced mushrooms
- 3 ounces sliced pepperoni
- 3/4 cup pizza sauce
- 2 1/4 cup shredded mozzarella cheese
- 1 teaspoon dried oregano

Directions:
1. Preheat oven to 300°F.
2. Drizzle a 13-by-18-inch rimmed baking sheet. Cook cream cheese keto crust as stated above until crust is golden brown.
3. Remove crust from the oven and increase oven temperature to 450°F.
4. Spread baked keto crust with olive oil and pizza sauce.
5. Sprinkle with mozzarella, top with mushrooms and pepperoni, and season with oregano.
6. Bake for 10 minutes. Slice and serve.

Italian Pizzas

Regina Pizza

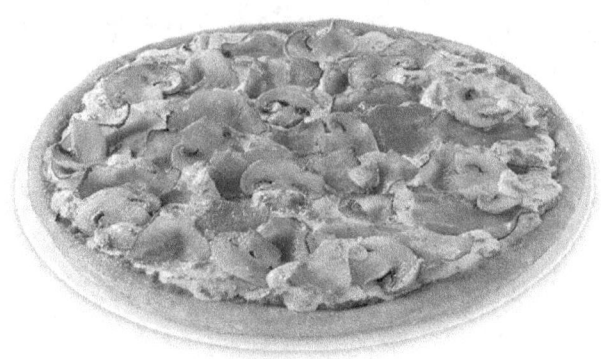

Nutrients per 100 g:
- Total Carbohydrates – 2.6 g
- Fat – 21.6 g
- Protein – 18.1 g
- Calories – 275.1

Ingredients:
- 1/3 cup your favorite pizza sauce
- 2 cups thinly sliced fresh mushrooms
- 1 1/2 cups chopped ham
- 2 cups shredded mozzarella cheese
- 1 sliced tomato
- 1 ounce sliced black olives, drained

- 1 teaspoon dried oregano

Directions:
1. Place sliced mushrooms in a small microwave-safe bowl. Microwave on high power until mushrooms are tender (for 2 to 3 minutes). Drain mushrooms.
2. Cook cream cheese keto crust as stated above.
3. Remove crust from the oven and increase oven temperature to 450°F.
4. Spread baked keto crust with pizza sauce and sprinkle with oregano.
5. Add the tomato, mozzarella, ham, mushrooms, and olives.
6. Bake until cheese is melted. Serve hot.

Margherita Pizza

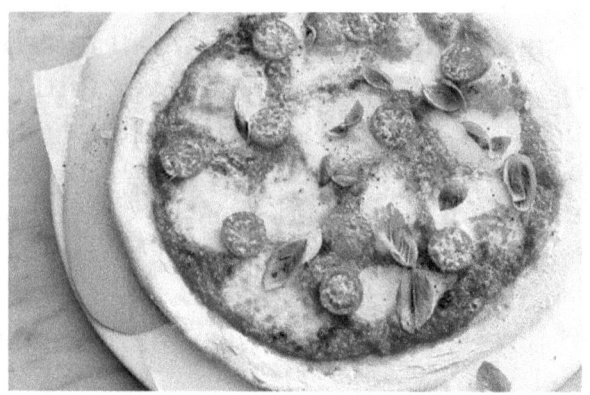

Nutrients per 100 g:
- Total Carbohydrates – 4.8 g
- Fat – 23.3 g
- Protein – 15.7 g
- Calories – 288.6

Ingredients:
- 1 tablespoon olive oil
- 2 cloves garlic, finely chopped
- 1/4 cup pizza sauce
- 8 oz. mozzarella cheese
- 2 tomatoes, sliced
- fresh basil
- fresh ground pepper, to taste

Directions:

1. Combine the olive oil and chopped garlic in a small dish.
2. Cook cream cheese keto crust as stated above.
3. Remove crust from the oven and increase oven temperature to 450°F.
4. Spread baked keto crust with olive oil/garlic mixture.
5. Top with pizza sauce, mozzarella cheese slices, and tomato slices.
6. Bake until cheese is melted. Remove from the oven. Top with basil and pepper before serving.

Marinara Pizza

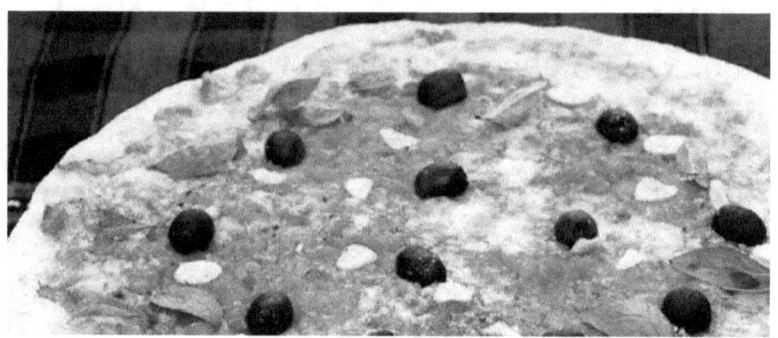

Nutrients per 100 g:
- Total Carbohydrates – 5.8 g
- Fat – 31.3 g
- Protein – 20.5 g
- Calories – 383.5

Ingredients:
- 2 tablespoons olive oil
- 3 cloves garlic, finely chopped
- 1/3 cup your favorite pizza sauce
- 1 1/2 cup mozzarella cheese, grated
- 100 g cherry tomatoes, halved
- 1/2 cup cooked salmon, chopped
- 1 ounce sliced black olives, drained
- 1 teaspoon dried oregano
- handful of fresh basil

Directions:
1. Mix olive oil and chopped garlic in a small dish.
2. Cook cream cheese keto crust as stated above.
3. Remove crust from the oven and increase oven temperature to 450°F.
4. Spread baked keto crust with olive oil/garlic mixture.
5. Spread tomato sauce, dried oregano, cherry tomatoes, salmon, and sliced black olives.
6. Top with mozzarella cheese and fresh basil.
7. Bake for 5 to 10 minutes until cheese is melted. Serve and enjoy!

Napoli Pizza with Anchovies

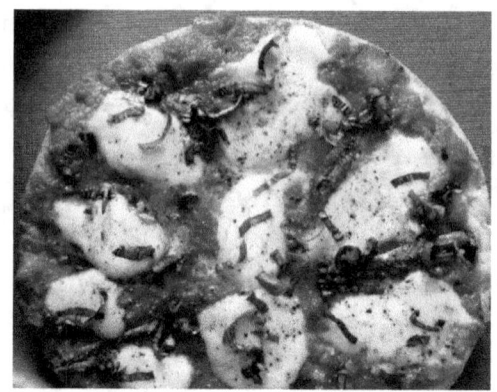

Nutrients per 100 g:
- Total Carbohydrates – 4.2 g
- Fat – 24.7 g
- Protein – 16.8 g
- Calories – 303.3

Ingredients:
- 2/3 cup pizza sauce
- 1 tablespoon olive oil
- 1 1/2 cups shredded mozzarella cheese
- 6 to 8 small anchovies
- 1 tablespoon salted capers, rinsed
- 1 teaspoon dried oregano
- pinch chili flakes (optional)

Directions:
1. Cook cream cheese keto crust as stated above.

2. Remove crust from the oven and increase oven temperature to 450°F.

3. Spread baked keto crust with olive oil and pizza sauce, leaving a 1-inch border.

4. Scatter the mozzarella cheese over pizza.

5. Arrange the anchovies and capers.

6. Sprinkle the oregano and chili flakes (if using) over the pizza.

7. Bake until cheese is melted. Slice and enjoy!

Capricciosa Pizza

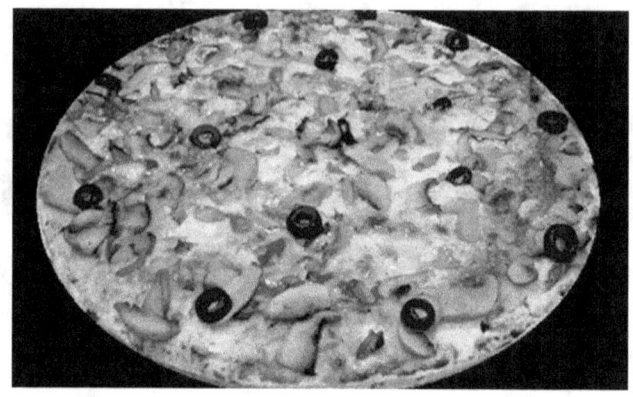

Nutrients per 100 g:
- Total Carbohydrates – 5.8 g
- Fat – 27.1 g
- Protein – 14 g
- Calories – 317.9

Ingredients:
- 1/2 cup puréed tomatoes (passata)
- white mushrooms in oil (champignons)
- 7 green olives, pitted
- 7 black olives, pitted
- 3 artichoke hearts, quartered
- 1 cup mozzarella cheese, shredded
- 1 tablespoon olive oil
- Salt to taste

- 1 teaspoon dried oregano

Directions:
1. Prepare tomato sauce by mixing puréed tomatoes with olive oil, dried oregano, and salt.
2. Cook cream cheese keto crust as stated above.
3. Remove crust from the oven and increase oven temperature to 450°F.
4. Spread baked keto crust with tomato sauce.
5. Arrange olives, mushrooms, artichokes, and mozzarella cheese over the pizza.
6. Place the pizza in the oven for 10 minutes until cheese is melted. Serve and enjoy!

Quattro Formaggi Pizza

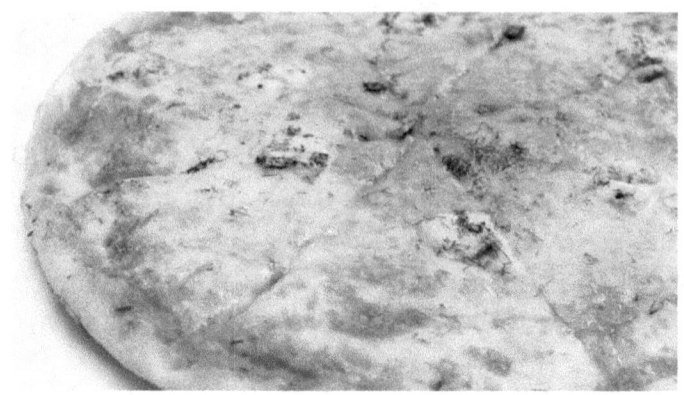

Nutrients per 100 g:
- Total Carbohydrates – 3.4 g
- Fat – 37.3 g
- Protein – 19 g
- Calories – 427.9

Ingredients:
- 1 1/4 cup full-fat mozzarella, shredded
- 7/8 cup gorgonzola cheese, crumbled
- 1 cup pecorino cheese, grated
- 7/8 cup ricotta cheese
- 2 garlic cloves, minced
- 1/2 teaspoon ground black pepper
- 1 teaspoon dried oregano

Directions:

1. Cook cream cheese keto crust as stated above.
2. Remove crust from the oven and increase oven temperature to 450°F.
3. Thinly slice the mozzarella and scatter evenly on the base, leaving the edges clear to about 3 to 4 cm (1½ inches), and then add garlic and oregano.
4. Spoon the ricotta in blobs over the mozzarella and place the Gorgonzola cubes randomly in places where there is no ricotta.
5. Scatter pecorino evenly over the top.
6. Season with black pepper and place the pizza in the oven for 3 to 5 minutes until cheese is melted. Remove from the oven. Serve and enjoy!

Quattro Stagioni Pizza

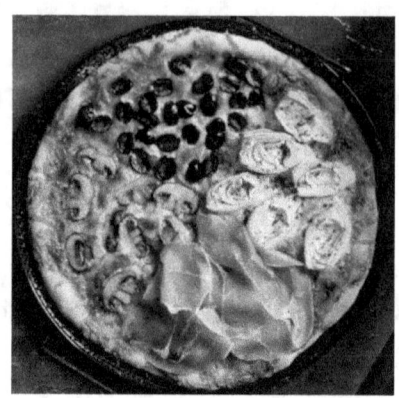

Nutrients per 100 g:

- Total Carbohydrates – 7.5 g
- Fat – 27.4 g
- Protein – 17 g
- Calories – 340.4

Ingredients:
- 2/3 cup pizza sauce
- 1 sliced tomato
- 2 oz. sliced mushrooms
- 1 1/2 cups mozzarella cheese, grated
- 3 artichoke hearts, quartered
- 1/3 cup black olives

- 2 oz. salami, sliced
- 2 teaspoons olive oil
- 2 garlic cloves, chopped
- A handful of fresh basil
- Ground black pepper to taste

Directions:
1. Fry the mushrooms in olive oil over medium heat until mushrooms are tender. Remove to cool.
2. Cook cream cheese keto crust as stated above.
3. Remove crust from the oven and increase oven temperature to 450°F.
4. Spread baked keto crust with pizza sauce, mozzarella cheese, and garlic.
5. Top one-quarter of the pizza with salami. Sprinkle with ground black pepper.
6. Top another quarter of the pizza with artichoke hearts and olives.
7. Top a third quarter with mushroom mixture and remaining quarter with tomato.
8. Sprinkle with snipped basil and bake until cheese is melted. Top with fresh basil. Serve.

Boscaiola Pizza

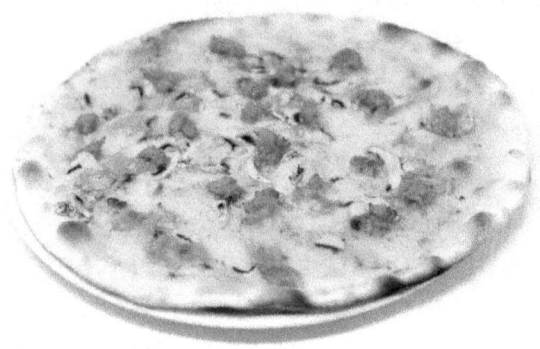

Nutrients per 100 g:
- Total Carbohydrates – 2.2 g
- Fat – 38.2 g
- Protein – 27.6 g
- Calories – 460

Ingredients:
- 1/2-pound sweet Italian sausages, meat removed from the casings
- 2 teaspoons extra-virgin olive oil
- 2 cups shredded mozzarella
- 2 cups sliced mushrooms
- 1 thinly sliced onion
- 2 garlic cloves, minced
- 2 tablespoons finely chopped flat-leaf parsley

- Ground black pepper to taste

Directions:
1. Pour on the olive oil in a large skillet and heat it. Add sausage, mushrooms, and onion to the skillet and cook for 7-10 minutes. Set aside to cool.
2. Cook cream cheese keto crust as stated above.
3. Remove crust from the oven and increase oven temperature to 450°F.
4. Spread baked keto crust with mozzarella cheese and garlic.
5. Top with cooked sausage, mushrooms, onion mixture, and chopped flat-leaf parsley.
6. Bake for 5 to 10 minutes until cheese is melted. Serve and enjoy!

Keto – bread

Bread contains cellulose. Why is cellulose healthy?

It lowers blood cholesterol and blood pressure, stimulates digestion, speeds up metabolism, removes toxins from the body, promotes cell renewal and helps maintain youth. At the same time, it quickly causes a feeling of satiety.

The Keto diet uses bread, which contains the minimum amount of carbohydrates and has other beneficial properties.

Sandwiches

Almond Buns

8 servings
Nutrients per 100 g:
- Total Carbohydrates – 6.1 g
- Fat – 42.6 g
- Protein – 17.5 g
- Calories – 484.9

Nutrients per serving (2 buns):

- Total Carbohydrates – 3.05 g
- Fat – 22.8 g
- Protein – 8.75 g
- Calories – 242.45

Ingredients:
- 90 g almond flour
- 50 g unsalted butter
- 2 eggs
- 1 teaspoon baking soda
- 1/2 teaspoon citric acid powder
- Salt (optional)
- Sesame (optional)
- Herbs (optional)

Directions:

1. Melt the butter in the microwave.

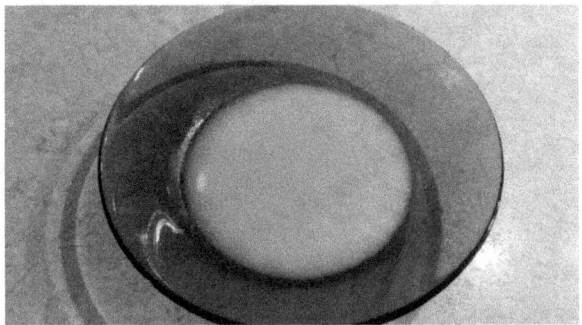

2. Add flour, eggs, salt (optional), herbs (optional), and mix with a spoon until smooth.

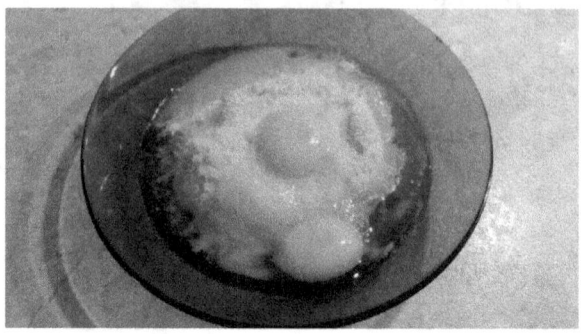

3. Preheat oven to 400°F.

4. Pound the citric acid powder in the saucer with a spoon until a homogeneous powder and mix with baking soda. Add the mixture to the dough and mix with a spoon.

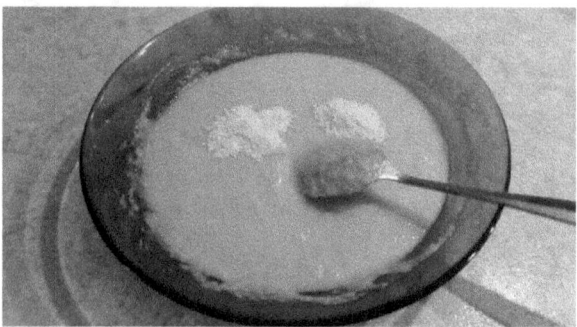

5. Fill 8 paper or silicone baking molds (3-inches diameter) with the dough. Sprinkle with sesame seeds (optional).

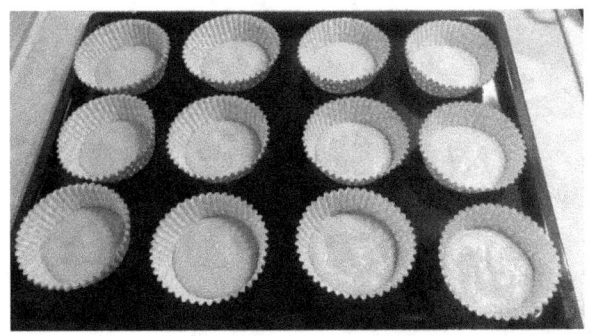

6. Bake for 10 minutes. Turn off the oven and leave the buns for another 5 minutes.

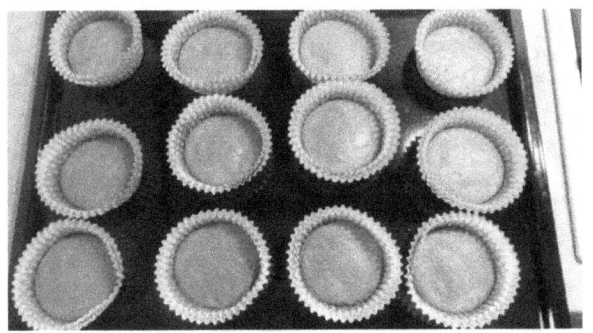

7. Cook sandwiches with pleasure!

Hamburger

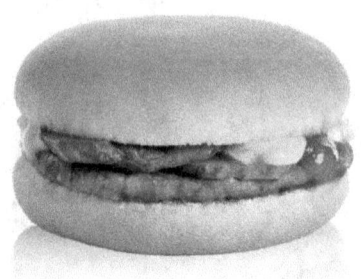

4 servings
Nutrients per serving:
- Total Carbohydrates – 8.2 g
- Fat – 32.5 g
- Protein – 21 g
- Calories – 396.1

Ingredients:
- 8 almond buns
- 1/2 pound ground beef
- Salt
- 4 tablespoons ketchup
- 2 teaspoons prepared mustard
- 2 teaspoons finely minced onion
- 4 dill pickle slices

Directions:

1. Cook 8 almond buns as stated above.
2. Roll the ground beef into 4 balls and then press it flat on wax paper (about 3 inches wide).
3. Cook the burger in the pan for 2-5 minutes per side. Salt both sides during the cooking.
4. On the top of one bun, spread the ketchup, mustard, and onion, in that order, and top with the pickle slice.
5. Put the beef patty on the bottom of another bun and slap both buns together.
6. Preheat the burger in the oven for 5 minutes (350 F) or microwave them on high for 10 to 15 seconds, if needed. Serve and enjoy!

Cheeseburger

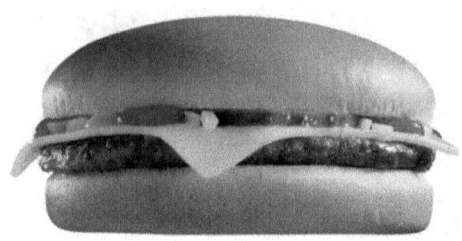

4 servings

Nutrients per serving:
- Total Carbohydrates – 8.8 g
- Fat – 42 g
- Protein – 29.6 g
- Calories – 518

Ingredients:
- 3/4 pounds ground beef
- 3 tablespoons salt
- 1 teaspoon black pepper
- 1/4 teaspoon onion powder
- 1/8 teaspoon garlic powder
- 4 American cheese slices
- 8 slices dill pickles
- 4 tablespoons chopped onion, soaked in cold water
- Mustard, to garnish
- Ketchup, to garnish
- 8 almond buns

Directions:

1. Cook 8 almond buns as stated above.
2. Blend the meat in a large bowl.
3. Combine salt, black pepper, onion and garlic powder in a separate bowl.
4. Roll the ground beef into 4 balls and then press it flat on wax paper (about 3 inches wide).
5. Heat a large, nonstick griddle to high. Cook burgers, turning once, for 6 to 8 minutes total until browned on both sides, remembering to season heavily.
6. Put the burgers on the top of 4 buns and add a slice of American cheese to each one.
7. Drain the onion thoroughly.
8. Garnish with ketchup and mustard. Place 2 slices of pickles on top.
9. Top the burger with the onion and other 4 buns. Serve hot and enjoy!

Classic Burger

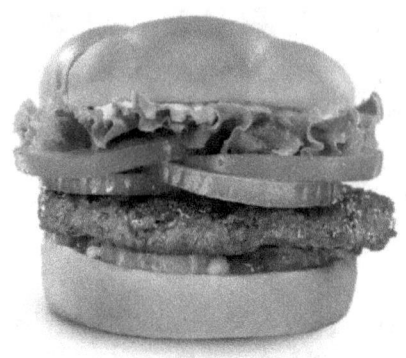

4 servings

Nutrients per serving:

- Total Carbohydrates – 8.8 g
- Fat – 45.8 g
- Protein – 28.6 g
- Calories – 548.8

Ingredients:

- 8 almond buns
- 3/4 pound ground beef
- 1 egg
- 1/4 teaspoon pepper
- 1/2 teaspoon salt
- 1 or 2 cloves garlic, minced
- 1/4 cup mayonnaise
- 1/4 cup ketchup

- 4 iceberg lettuce leaves, rinsed and crisped
- 1 firm-ripe tomato, cored and thinly sliced
- 4 thin slices red onion

Directions:
1. Combine ground beef, egg, garlic, salt, and pepper. Make four equal portions and shape each into a patty about 3 inches wide.
2. Cook burgers for 6 to 8 minutes, turning once until browned on both sides.
3. Cook 8 almond buns as stated above.
4. Spread mayonnaise and ketchup on 4 buns.
5. Place lettuce, tomato, burger, onion, and salt and pepper to taste. Set another 4 buns on top. Serve.

Breakfast Sandwich

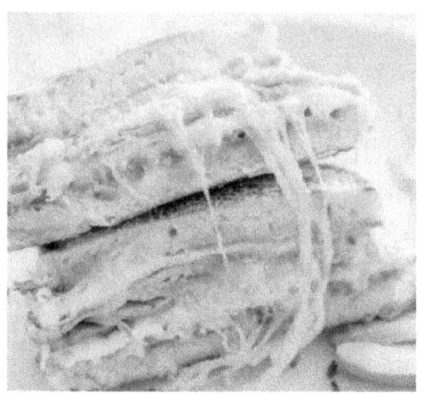

4 servings
Nutrients per serving:
- Total Carbohydrates – 5.1 g
- Fat – 57.2 g
- Protein – 41.6 g
- Calories – 668.2

Ingredients:
- 8 almond buns
- 8 eggs
- 4 slices of ham
- 1 1/2 cups finely shredded Mexican cheese
- salt and pepper to taste
- 8 slices of bacon

Directions:
1. Cook 8 almond buns as stated above.
2. For one sandwich heat a large non-stick pan over medium heat.
3. Cook 2 slices of bacon side by side on the pan, then crack 2 eggs on the bacon and break the yolks with a spatula.
4. Sprinkle tops of each egg with salt and pepper to taste, and 1/8 cup of shredded cheese. Place 2 buns over the eggs and lightly press on the tops with a spatula.
5. Turn the sandwich (egg-side-up). Top with ham and 1/8 cup of shredded cheese one half of your sandwich. Fold the sandwich together and serve.

Bauru (Brazilian Roast Beef Sandwich)

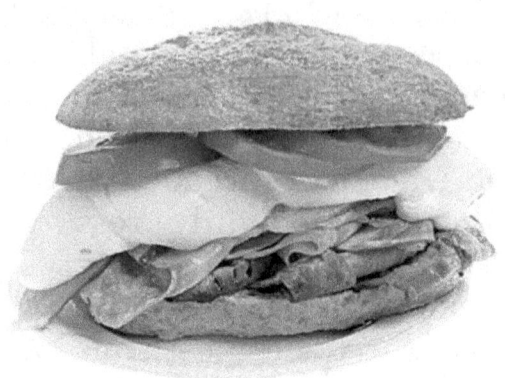

4 servings

Nutrients per serving:
- Total Carbohydrates – 5.6 g
- Fat – 33.7 g
- Protein – 24.2 g
- Calories – 418.2

Ingredients:
- 8 almond buns
- 16 slices deli roast beef
- 4 slices tomato
- 8 dill pickle chips
- 8 (1/4"-thick) slices mozzarella

Directions:

1. Cook 8 almond buns as stated above.
2. Heat oven to 350°.
3. Place roast beef, pickles, mozzarella, and tomato on the 4 buns. Cover with another 4 buns and place on a baking sheet.
4. Bake about 5-7 minutes until cheese is melted. Serve hot.

Almond Bread

12 servings

Nutrients per 100 g:
- Total Carbohydrates – 6.1 g
- Fat – 42.6 g
- Protein – 17.5 g
- Calories – 484.9

Ingredients:
- 90 g almond flour
- 50 g unsalted butter
- 2 eggs
- 1 teaspoon baking soda
- 1/2 teaspoon citric acid powder
- Salt (optional)
- Sesame (optional)
- Herbs (optional)

Directions:
1. Melt the butter in the microwave.
2. Add flour, eggs, salt (optional), herbs (optional), and mix with a spoon until smooth.
3. Preheat oven to 400°F.
4. Pound the citric acid powder in the saucer with a spoon until a homogeneous powder and mix with baking soda. Add the mixture to the dough and mix with a spoon.
5. Fill a 3x4-inch baking form with the dough. Sprinkle with sesame seeds (optional).

6. Bake for 20 minutes. Turn off the oven and leave the buns for another 10 minutes.

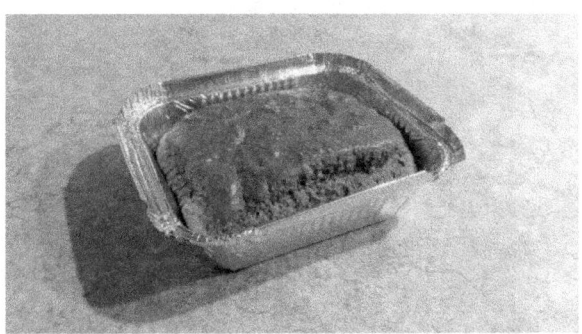

7. Cook sandwiches with pleasure!

Avocado BLT

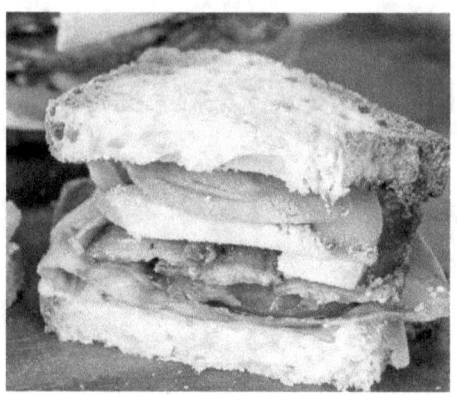

4 servings

Nutrients per serving:
- Total Carbohydrates – 5.33 g
- Fat – 42.8 g
- Protein – 18.45 g
- Calories – 470.9

Ingredients:
- 8 slices almond bread
- 1 large tomato sliced
- 4 lettuce leaves
- 1/2 avocado sliced
- 4 tablespoons mayonnaise
- 12 slices bacon cooked

Directions:
1. Cook almond bread as stated above and slice it. 8 slices are needed.
2. Heat a large, nonstick skillet too high to cook the bacon. Fry it for 2-3 minutes until browned on both sides.
3. Spread 4 tablespoons of mayonnaise on 8 slices of bread.
4. On top of 4 slices, place lettuce leaves, slices of tomatoes, 3 slices of bacon, then avocado slices and another 4 slices of bread. Serve and enjoy!

Tuna Sandwich

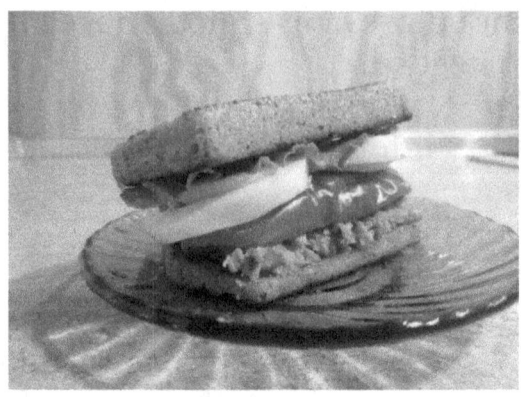

4 servings

Nutrients per serving:

- Total Carbohydrates – 5.3 g
- Fat – 32.4 g
- Protein – 26.9 g
- Calories – 412.7

Ingredients:

- 8 slices almond bread
- 2 cans tuna (8-oz.), drained
- 3 tablespoons pitted olives, chopped
- 2 tablespoons olive oil
- 1 teaspoon paprika
- salt, to taste
- 2 hard-boiled egg, sliced
- 1 roasted pepper, cut into 4 parts
- 4 lettuce leaves

Directions:
1. Preheat the oven to 425°F.
2. Clean and dry the pepper and place into an oven safe dish or a roasting pan.
3. Cook about 30 minutes until peppers are soft and browned in spots, turning them a couple of times during cooking.
4. Remove from oven and cover or wrap in a paper bag. Let cool about 15-20 minutes. Peel it, remove the stem, cut the pepper lengthwise into 4 strips and remove seeds.
5. Cook almond bread as stated above and slice it. 8 slices are needed.
6. Mix tuna, olives, olive oil, paprika, and salt in a bowl.
7. Set 1/4 mixture on bread.
8. Top with 1 piece of roasted pepper, 2-3 slices of egg, lettuce, and another slice of bread. Enjoy!

Cheese Dreams Sandwich

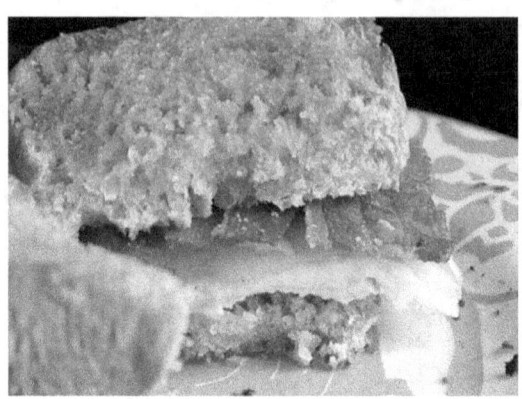

4 servings

Nutrients per serving:
- Total Carbohydrates – 3.7 g
- Fat – 58.7 g
- Protein – 28.5 g
- Calories – 650

Ingredients:
- 8 slices almond bread
- 8 slices bacon, diced
- 1/4 cup mayonnaise
- 2 tablespoons soft butter or margarine
- 2 cups grated sharp Cheddar cheese
- 2 teaspoons grated onion
- 1 pinch cayenne pepper

Directions:

1. Cook almond bread as stated above and slice it. 8 slices are needed.
2. Fry bacon until crisp; let cool, then dice.
3. Preheat the oven to 350F.
4. Mix mayonnaise and butter. Combine cheese, onion and cayenne pepper until well blended. Gently stir in bacon.
5. Spread mixture on slices of bread.
6. Place on buttered baking sheet and bake until cheese is melted. Serve hot.

Tuscan Tuna Sandwich

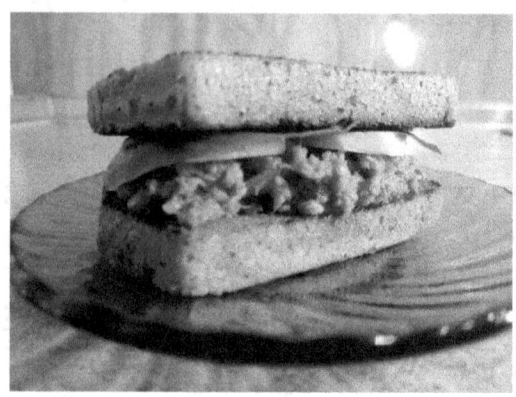

4 servings

Nutrients per serving:
- Total Carbohydrates – 6.2 g
- Fat – 39.5 g
- Protein – 28.3 g
- Calories – 488.8

Ingredients:
- 8 slices almond bread
- 2 (8-oz.) cans tuna, drained
- 1/2 cup roughly chopped sun-dried tomatoes
- 4 tablespoons olive oil
- 3 tablespoons roughly chopped capers
- salt, to taste

- ground black pepper, to taste
- 4 slices mozzarella cheese
- basil leaves

Directions:

1. Cook almond bread as stated above and slice it. 8 slices are needed.

2. Mix tuna, sun-dried tomatoes, olive oil, capers, salt, and pepper in a bowl.

3. Place mixture on the 4 slices of bread.

4. Serve with basil leaves and sliced mozzarella. Top with remaining 4 slices.

All-American Club Sandwich

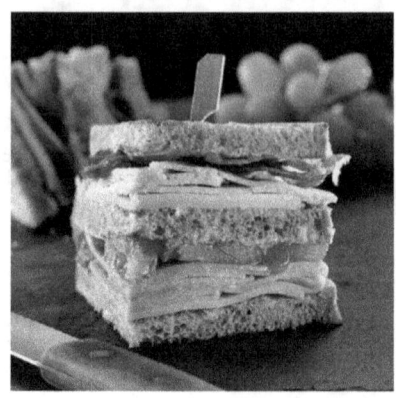

8 servings

Nutrients per serving:

- Total Carbohydrates – 5.9 g
- Fat – 32.5 g
- Protein – 18.4 g
- Calories – 376.4

Ingredients:

- 1/3 cup mayonnaise
- 2 tablespoons Dijon-style mustard
- 12 slices almond bread
- 1/2 pound deli turkey breast, thinly sliced
- 8 slices cooked bacon
- 1/2 pound thinly sliced deli ham
- 8 (3/4-ounce) slices deli American cheese
- 8 slices tomato
- 8 lettuce leaves

Directions:
1. Cook almond bread as stated above.
2. Mix mayonnaise and mustard in a bowl.
3. Spread a teaspoon of mayonnaise mixture on the side of each almond bread slice.
4. Take a slice of bread (mayonnaise-side up) and lay a lettuce leaf, a slice of cheese, 2 ounces of ham, 2 slices of tomato, a slice of bread (mayonnaise-side down), spread a teaspoon of mayonnaise on bread.
5. Then place on a top of each sandwich a slice of cheese, 2 ounces of turkey, 2 slices of bacon, a lettuce leaf, and a slice of bread (mayonnaise-side down).
6. Cut into triangles. Secure with toothpicks. Serve and enjoy!

Ham and Cheese Sandwich

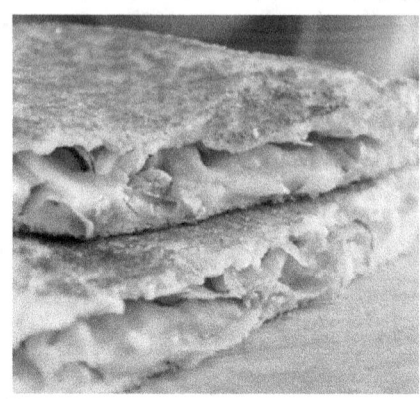

4 servings
Nutrients per serving:
- Total Carbohydrates – 3.7 g
- Fat – 41 g
- Protein – 19.9 g
- Calories – 449

Ingredients:
- 8 slices almond bread
- 8 teaspoons butter
- 8 slices Swiss cheese
- 8 thin slices deli ham
- 4 teaspoons mayonnaise
- 4 teaspoons whole grain mustard

Directions:
1. Cook almond bread as stated above and slice it. 8 slices are needed.
2. Preheat a skillet over medium-high heat.
3. Spread one side of 8 slices of bread with a teaspoon of butter.
4. Place 4 slices of bread, butter-side down in the hot skillet.
5. Top with Swiss cheese and ham.
6. Spread the unbuttered sides of another 4 slices of bread with mayonnaise and mustard. Place them, butter-side up on top of the sandwiches.
7. Cook until the sandwiches are golden brown and the cheese is melted (about 3 minutes per side).

Turkey Melt Sandwich

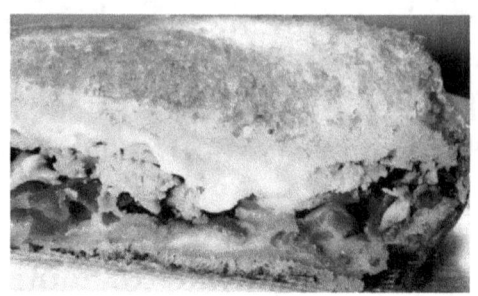

4 servings
Nutrients per serving:
- Total Carbohydrates – 6.25 g
- Fat – 46.58 g
- Protein – 34.55 g
- Calories – 572

Ingredients:
- 8 slices almond bread
- 1/2 lb. turkey lunch meat
- 4 tablespoons mayonnaise
- 8 tomato slices
- 8 cooked bacon slices
- 8 provolone cheese slices or your favorite cheese

Directions:

1. Cook almond bread as stated above and slice it. 8 slices are needed.
2. Preheat oven to 400 degrees.
3. Lightly toast your bread slices.
4. Spread 1 tablespoon of mayonnaise on a piece of toast.
5. Layer 1/4 lb. of turkey lunch meat, 2 tomato slices, 2 pieces of bacon and 2 slices of cheese on top of toast.
6. Place another slice of bread on top and place on baking sheet; repeat steps until all sandwiches are done.
7. Place the sandwiches in the oven for 5-10 minutes until cheese is melted. Serve and enjoy!

Almond Hot-Dog Buns

4 servings

Nutrients per 100 g:
- Total Carbohydrates – 6.1 g
- Fat – 42.6 g
- Protein – 17.5 g
- Calories – 484.9

Nutrients per serving:
- Total Carbs – 3.05 g
- Fat – 22.8 g
- Protein – 8.75 g
- Calories – 242.45

Ingredients:
- 90 g almond flour
- 50 g unsalted butter
- 2 eggs
- 1 teaspoon baking soda
- 1/2 teaspoon citric acid powder
- Salt (optional)
- Sesame (optional)
- Herbs (optional)

Directions:
1. Melt the butter in the microwave.
2. Add flour, eggs, salt (optional), herbs (optional), and mix with a spoon until smooth.
3. Preheat oven to 400°F.

4. Pound the citric acid powder in the saucer with a spoon until a homogeneous powder and mix with baking soda. Add the mixture to the dough and mix with a spoon.

5. Fill 4 paper or silicone baking molds for hot-dog buns with the dough. Sprinkle with sesame seeds (optional).

6. Bake for 15 minutes. Turn off the oven and leave the buns for another 8 minutes.

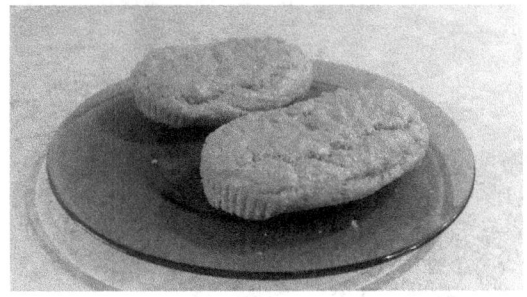

7. Cook sandwiches with pleasure!

Medianoche Sandwich

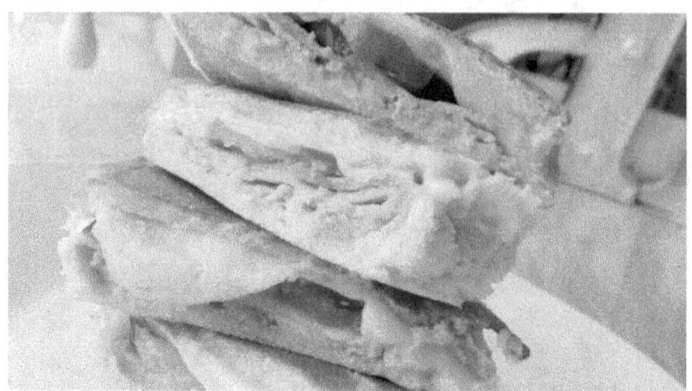

4 servings

Nutrients per serving:

- Total Carbohydrates – 11.8 g
- Fat – 88.6 g
- Protein – 45.1 g
- Calories – 1017.7

Ingredients:

- 4 almond hot-dog buns
- 1/2 cup mayonnaise
- 1/4 cup prepared mustard
- 1/4 pound thinly sliced cooked ham
- 1/2 pound thinly sliced cooked pork
- 1/2 pound sliced Swiss cheese
- 1/2 cup dill pickle slices
- 2 tablespoons butter, melted

Directions:
1. Cook 4 almond hot-dog buns as stated above.
2. Split the buns in half, and spread mustard and mayonnaise onto the cut sides.
3. Melt butter and brush the top of each sandwich.
4. Place equal portions of Swiss cheese, ham, pork, and a few pickles on each sandwich.
5. Put the tops of the buns onto the sandwiches.
6. Heat a large skillet over medium-high heat, and press the sandwiches down using a sturdy plate or another skillet. Flip them once for even browning. Serve hot.

Gerber Sandwich

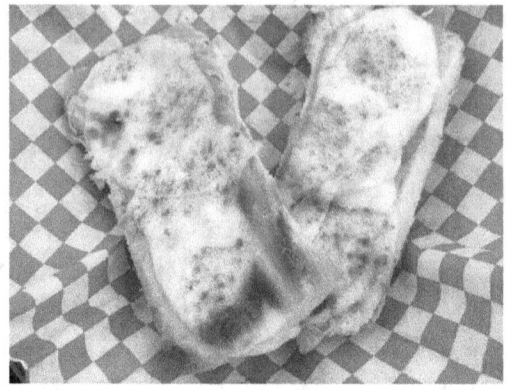

4 servings
Nutrients per serving:
- Total Carbohydrates – 5.8 g
- Fat – 41.2 g
- Protein – 22.9 g
- Calories – 475.5

Ingredients:
- 4 almond hot-dog buns
- 8 teaspoons butter
- 4 cloves of garlic, minced
- 8 slices of ham
- 8 slices Provolone cheese
- Paprika

Directions:
1. Cook 4 almond hot-dog buns as stated above.
2. Slice almond hot-dog buns in half.
3. Preheat oven to 350 degrees.
4. In a small dish, mash garlic with butter. Spread on almond buns.
5. Top with ham and cheese.
6. Sprinkle a touch of paprika.
7. Bake until cheese is melted (for 5-10 minutes). Serve immediately.

Bacon Barbecue Dog

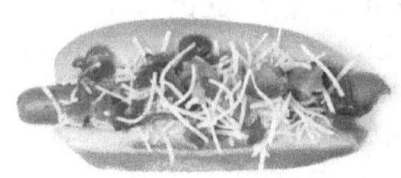

4 servings
Nutrients per serving:
- Total Carbohydrates – 6.9 g
- Fat – 54 g
- Protein – 26 g
- Calories – 613.2

Ingredients:
- 4 almond hot-dog buns
- 4 slices bacon
- 4 hot dogs
- 1/8 cup barbecue sauce
- 4 ounces Cheddar, grated (1 cup)

Directions:
1. Cook 4 almond hot-dog buns as stated above.
2. Heat a large skillet. Fry bacon over medium heat until crisp. Let cool, then crumble.

3. Cook the hot dogs by following the package directions.
4. Place a hot dog in each bun.
5. Top with the barbecue sauce, bacon, and Cheddar. Serve and enjoy!

Flax- bread

Bread from flax not only tastes like bread but also contains omega- 3 and cellulose (fiber).

It should be remembered that this kind of bread might have a laxative effect, which leads to significant water loss. Therefore, it is necessary to replenish your water balance in a timely manner.

Nutrients per 100 g:
- Total Carbohydrates – 5.5 g
- Fat – 30.6 g
- Protein – 18.4 g
- Calories – 370

Ingredients:
- 100 g flax seeds
- 1 egg
- 50 g milk
- salt
- Provencal herbs

Directions:

1. Preheat oven to 400°F.

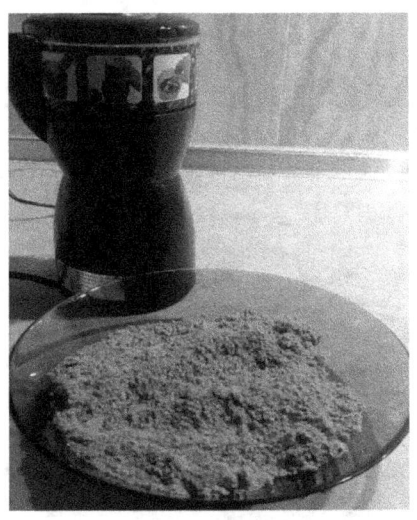

2. Grind flax seeds in a grinder.

3. Add herbs, salt, egg, milk to seeds. Mix with a whisk. Set aside for 10-15 minutes to swell the seeds.

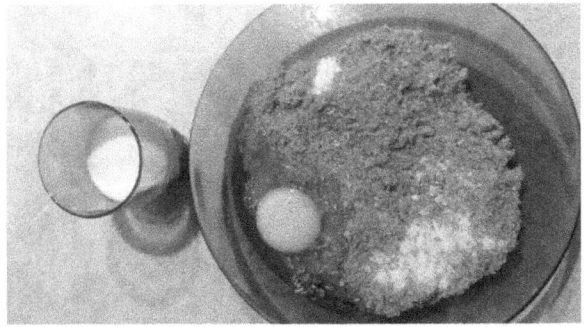

4. Fill a 3x4-inch baking form with the dough.
5. Bake for about 20 minutes until bread are fully cooked or toothpick inserted comes out clean. Turn off the oven and leave the bread for another 15 minutes.

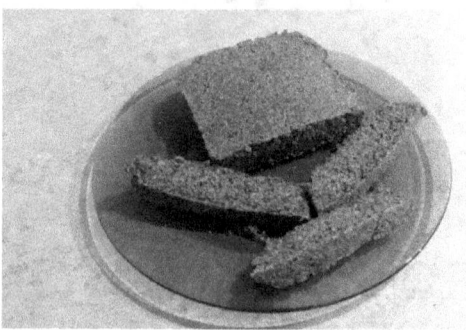

Keto Peanut Butter Buns

Nutrients per 100 g:
- Total Carbohydrates – 20.8 g
- Fat – 47.1 g
- Protein – 24.7 g
- Calories – 568.4

Ingredients:
- 250 g natural peanut butter
- 3 large eggs
- 1 teaspoon vinegar
- 1/2 teaspoon baking soda
- Salt

Directions:
1. Preheat oven to 350°F.

2. In a medium bowl, combine all the ingredients. Hand whisk or use mixer to mix until everything is smooth.

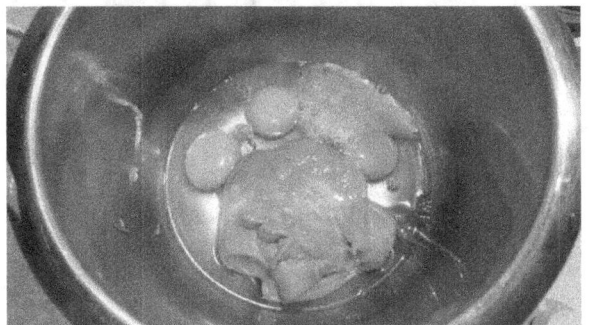

3. Fill 8 paper or silicone baking molds (3-inches diameter) with the dough.

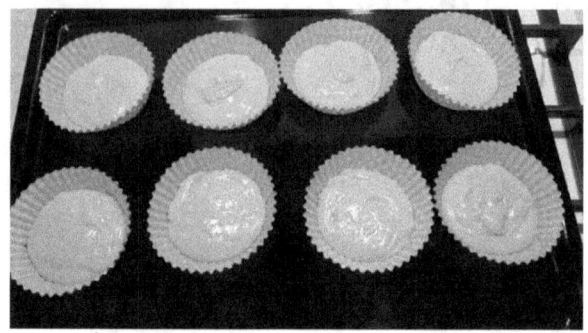

4. Bake for about 20 minutes until buns are fully cooked or toothpick inserted comes out clean. Turn off the oven and leave the buns for another 10 minutes.

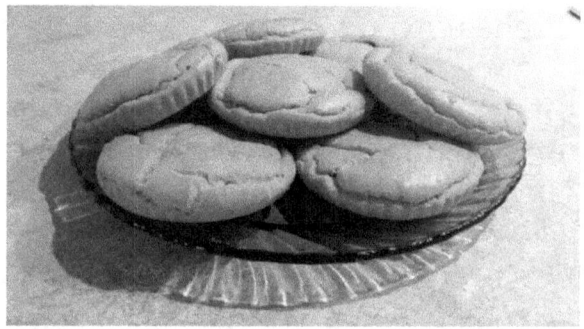

Pates

Pates and other dishes that contain large amounts of fat help to stick to a chosen Keto diet plan. You can choose any keto bread presented in this book. A variety of keto bread will allow you to eat full-fat foods with pleasure.

To calculate the energy value, you need:
1. weigh the bread and pate;
2. recalculate nutritional value by weight;
3. add carbohydrates, fats, proteins and calories of bread and carbohydrates, fats, proteins and calories of pate.

Simple Smoked Salmon Pate

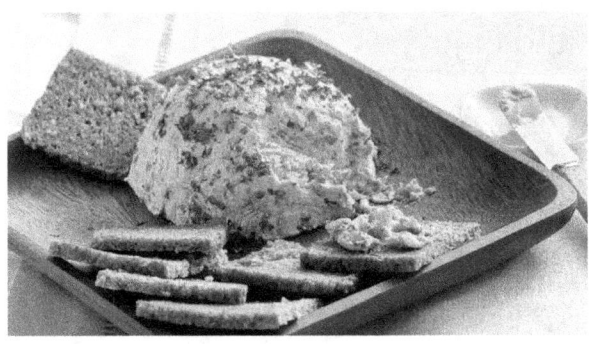

4 servings
Nutrients per 100 g:
- Total Carbohydrates – 2.9 g

- Fat – 28.6 g
- Protein – 13.6 g
- Calories – 323.3

Ingredients:
- 3 1/2 oz. full-fat cream cheese
- 3 1/2 oz. fat crème Fraiche
- 7 oz. smoked salmon
- 1 lemon, zest only, finely grated
- 1/2 lemon, juice only
- 1 tablespoon creamed horseradish
- 2 tablespoons finely chopped, fresh dill

Directions:
1. Process all the ingredients in the food processor. The pate should have some texture.
2. Taste to check the seasoning. It may also need more lemon juice or salt.
3. Serve and enjoy.

Easy Chicken Liver Pate

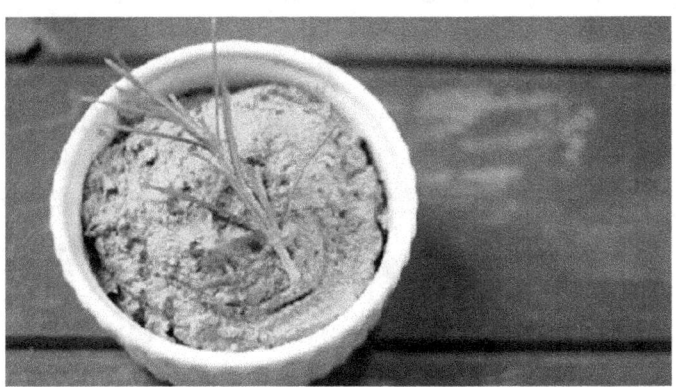

4 servings

Nutrients per 100 g:
- Total Carbohydrates – 1.6 g
- Fat – 34.1 g
- Protein – 19.3 g
- Calories – 390.8

Ingredients:
- 1/2 lb. chicken livers, trimmed
- 3 1/2 oz. butter, melted
- 1 fl. oz. double cream
- 1/2 tablespoon Armagnac or brandy
- Salt, to taste
- Ground black pepper, to taste

Directions:

1. Heat a teaspoon of the melted butter in a heavy-based frying pan over medium heat.
2. Cook half the chicken livers for three minutes until the livers become pink in the middle and cooked on the outside.
3. Remove them to a dish and repeat with the rest of the livers.
4. Blend the chicken livers in a food processor until smooth.
5. Add the remaining melted butter, salt, pepper, and double cream and blend once more.
6. Pour in the Armagnac or brandy.
7. Refrigerate before serving.

Smoked Mackerel Pate

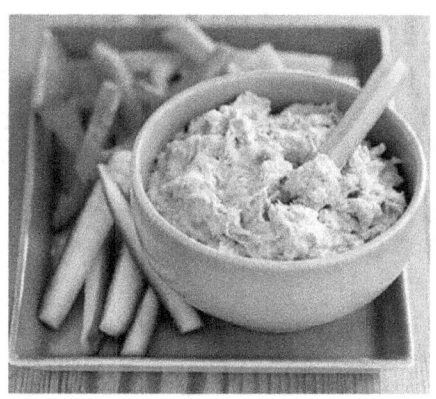

4 servings
Nutrients per 100 g:
- Total Carbohydrates – 5.6 g
- Fat – 19.7 g
- Protein – 23.3 g
- Calories – 296.9

Ingredients:
- 2 (160 g) smoked mackerel fillets, skinned and boned
- 5 oz. soured cream
- 4 oz. cottage cheese
- juice of half a lemon, or more
- grated nutmeg, to taste
- black pepper, to taste
- salt, to taste

- cayenne, to taste

Directions:
1. Pulse all the ingredients in a food processor (or in a blender) for a minute or so until smooth.
2. Season to taste with black pepper, nutmeg, and salt. Taste to check the seasoning. It may need more lemon juice.
3. Put into one large dish, cover with cling film and chill for two hours.
4. Sprinkle with a little cayenne and serve.

Bacon-Beef Liver Pate

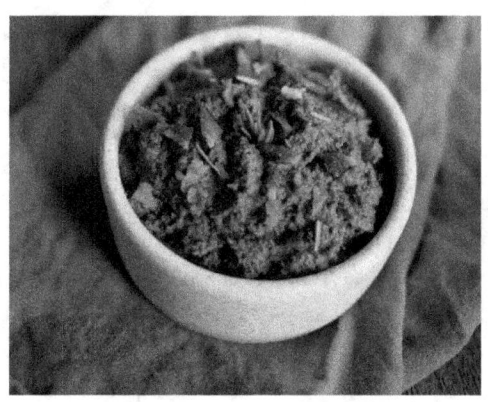

4 servings

Nutrients per 100 g:
- Total Carbohydrates – 2 g
- Fat – 23.4 g
- Protein – 13.8 g
- Calories – 272.8

Ingredients:
- 3 pieces uncured bacon
- 1/2 small onion, minced
- 2 cloves garlic, minced
- 1/2 pound grass-fed beef liver
- 1 tablespoon fresh rosemary, minced
- 1 tablespoon fresh thyme, minced
- 1/4 cup coconut oil, melted

- Salt, to taste

Directions:

1. Cook the bacon slices until crispy. Transfer the slices to a plate and leave them to cool. Reserve the grease.
2. Sprinkle the liver with the herbs and set aside.
3. Using the bacon grease, cook the onion for 3-5 minutes on medium-high.
4. Then add the minced garlic and continue to cook for a minute.
5. Add the liver. Cook it until no longer pink in the middle (about 5 minutes per side).
6. Place the liver and vegetables into a food processor or a blender with the coconut oil and salt. Blend until smooth. Add more coconut oil if too thick.
7. Cut the bacon strips into little bits and combine with the pate in a bowl. Serve with some fresh herbs.

Red Salmon Pate

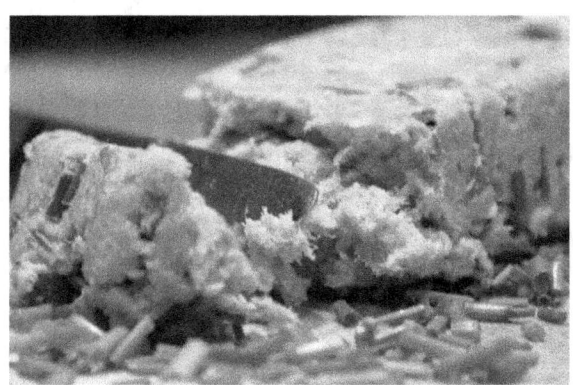

4 servings
Nutrients per 100 g:
- Total Carbohydrates – 3.6 g
- Fat – 24.9 g
- Protein – 15.1 g
- Calories – 293.2

Ingredients:
- 1/2 can (7 oz.) salmon, drained, flaked and bones removed
- 1/2 package (8 oz.) full-fat cream cheese, softened
- 1/2 teaspoon prepared horseradish
- 1/2 tablespoon lemon juice
- 1 teaspoon grated onion
- 1/2 tablespoon chopped fresh parsley

- 1/4 cup chopped pecans (optional)

Directions:
1. Combine all the ingredients in a bowl. Mix well.
2. Put into individual serving plates or a large dish. Be sure to cover with clingfilm.
3. Chill for two hours. Serve and enjoy.

Trout Pate

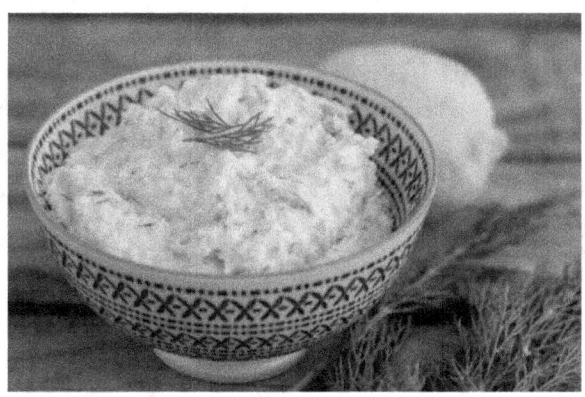

8 servings

Nutrients per 100 g:

- Total Carbohydrates – 0.9 g
- Fat – 18 g
- Protein – 13.6 g
- Calories – 225.5

Ingredients:

- 400 g hot smoked trout
- 75 g unsalted butter
- 170 ml carton soured cream
- 1 lemon, only juice
- Salt
- freshly ground black pepper

Directions:
1. Melt the butter in the microwave.
2. Beat in the butter, the cream, lemon juice, salt, and black pepper in a large bowl.
3. Check the fish for any bones and flake it into the bowl. Mix in gently to keep some texture.
4. Cover and chill the pate.
5. Let warm up at room temperature for 20 minutes before serving.

Duck Liver Pate

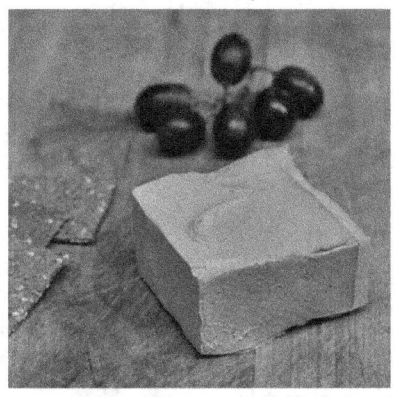

3 servings
Nutrients per 100 g:
- Total Carbohydrates – 5.1 g
- Fat – 42.8 g
- Protein – 11.2 g
- Calories – 447.1

Ingredients:
- 3 oz. duck liver, cut into pieces
- 1 large shallot, minced
- 2 oz. ghee
- herbs de Provence
- 1 clove garlic, peeled and crushed
- 1 teaspoon Cognac
- salt
- ground black pepper

Directions:
1. Cut the liver, sprinkle with the herbs de Provence and set aside.
2. Place ghee in a skillet, and cook the shallots over medium heat for a minute, stirring occasionally.
3. Add the liver and garlic, cook over medium to high heat for about 2 minutes, stirring occasionally. Season with salt and pepper.
4. Place the mixture into a blender, add the Cognac, and blend until smooth.
5. Cover, let cool, then chill. Serve and enjoy!

Sardine-Avocado Pate

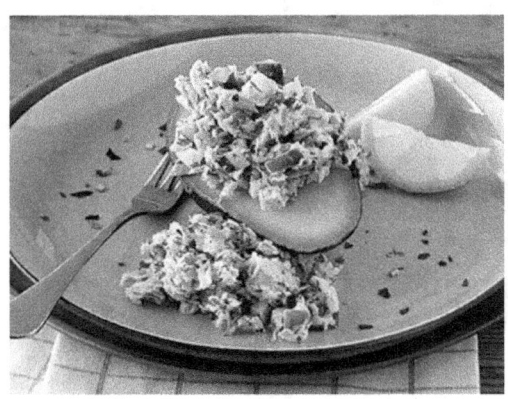

4 servings
Nutrients per 100 g:
- Total Carbohydrates – 4.5 g
- Fat – 20.8 g
- Protein – 9.2 g
- Calories – 233.7

Ingredients:
- 1 large avocado (5 1/4 oz.), seed removed and peeled
- 1 (3.2 oz.) tin sardines, drained
- 1 tablespoon mayonnaise
- 1 medium spring onion or bunch chives (0.5 oz.)
- 1 tablespoon fresh lemon juice
- 1/4 teaspoon turmeric powder
- 1/4 teaspoon salt

Directions:
1. Drain the sardines, check the fish for any bones and flake it into the bowl.
2. Halve the avocado, peel it, remove the seed, and scoop it to the bowl.
3. Then add turmeric powder, and mayonnaise and mix well.
4. Pulse the mixture in a food processor or a blender for a minute or so to desired consistency.
5. Add finely sliced spring onion (or chives), fresh lemon juice, season with salt and mix once more. Serve and enjoy.

Easy Duck Liver Pate

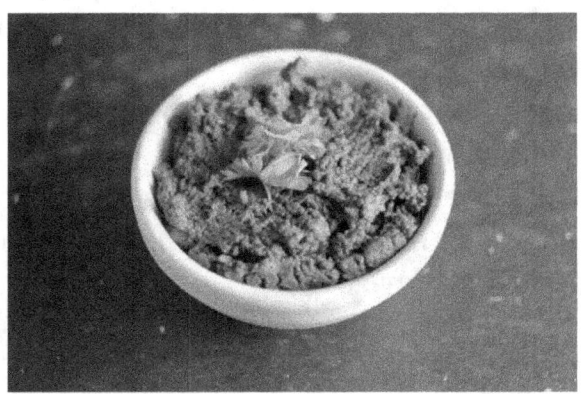

8 servings
Nutrients per 100 g:
- Total Carbohydrates – 3.3 g
- Fat – 30.4 g
- Protein – 15 g
- Calories – 350.8

Ingredients:
- 1 lb. Luv-a-Duck, duck livers
- 7 oz. butter, melted
- 50 ml double cream
- 1 tablespoon brandy
- sea salt
- freshly ground black pepper

Directions:

1. Heat a little of the melted butter into a heavy-based frying pan over medium heat.

2. Add half the duck livers and cook until well roasted. Put them to a plate and repeat with the rest of the livers.

3. Process the livers in a food processor for a minute or so until smooth.

4. Pour in the remaining butter, brandy, double cream, add salt and freshly ground black pepper and blend once more.

5. Taste to check the seasoning. Serve and enjoy.

Garlic Feta Pate

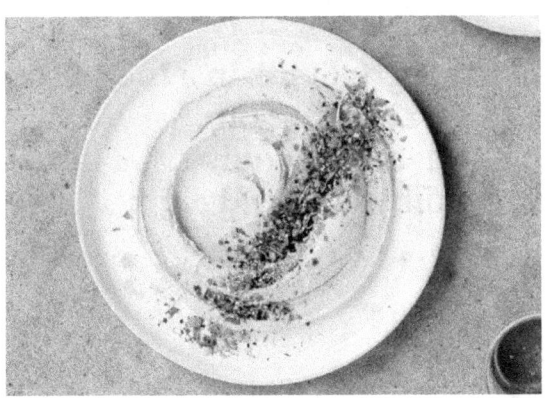

8 servings

Nutrients per 100 g:

- Total Carbohydrates – 4 g
- Fat – 34.3 g
- Protein – 7.1 g
- Calories – 349.4

Ingredients:

- fresh black pepper, ground, add to taste
- 1 dash hot pepper sauce, to flavor
- 1 tablespoon fresh chives, chopped
- 4 anchovy chopped fillets
- 6 tablespoons butter, softened
- 3/4 cup feta cheese (smashed)
- 1 (8 oz.) package cream cheese, softened

- 1/4 cup sour cream
- 2 cloves minced garlic

Directions:
1. Blend all the ingredients in a food processor or a blender. Pulse until smooth.
2. Taste to check the seasoning.
3. Cover and chill. Serve and enjoy.

Salmon and Cream Cheese Pate

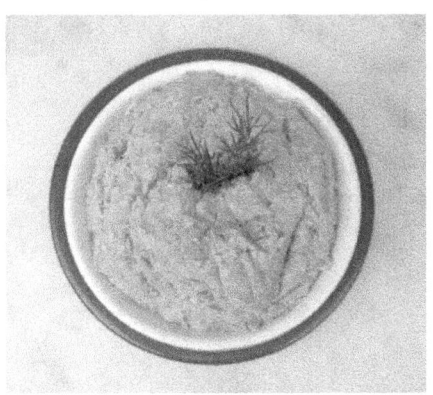

14 servings
Nutrients per 100 g:
- Total Carbohydrates – 2.5 g
- Fat – 11 g
- Protein – 18 g
- Calories – 182.4

Ingredients:
- 1 (14 1/2-oz.) can red salmon, drained
- 8 oz. soft cream cheese with chives and onions
- 2 teaspoons lemon juice
- 1/4 cup red bell pepper, chopped
- 1/2 teaspoon dried dill weed

Directions:
1. Line small bowl with clingfilm.

2. Drain the salmon, check the fish for any bones and flake it into the bowl.
3. Add the rest of the ingredients. Combine well.
4. Place into the lined bowl, press gently and cover.
5. Chill 1 to 2 hours.
6. Unmold pate onto a serving plate, remove plastic wrap and serve.

Pork-Pistachio Pate

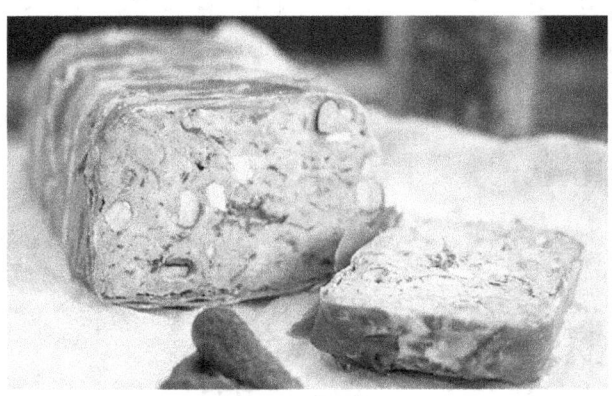

8 servings
Nutrients per 100 g:
- Total Carbohydrates – 3.1 g
- Fat – 32.2 g
- Protein – 17.9 g
- Calories – 374

Ingredients:
- 12 oz. ground pork
- 1 oz. fatback, cut into ½-inch pieces
- 2 oz. yellow onions, peeled and cut into quarters
- 2 small cloves garlic, smashed, peeled, and sliced
- 1 tablespoon brandy
- 1 teaspoon dried thyme

- 1/2 teaspoon dried oregano
- 1/2 teaspoon ground fennel seeds
- 1/2 teaspoon freshly ground black pepper
- Kosher salt
- 1 oz. shelled pistachio nuts

Directions:

1. Place ground pork, fatback, garlic, onion, seasonings in a food processor and process until smooth. Add brandy and salt.
2. Add the pistachio nuts and mix well.
3. Grease a 9-x-S-x-3-inch glass or ceramic loaf pan. Place the mixture into the pan. Smooth the surface with a spatula.
4. Cover tightly with plastic wrap. Microwave at full power for 7 minutes.
Prick the plastic to release steam.
5. Uncover and let to cool. Weight the plate with a foil-wrapped brick, when cool. Refrigerate overnight. Serve and enjoy.

Easy Liver Pate

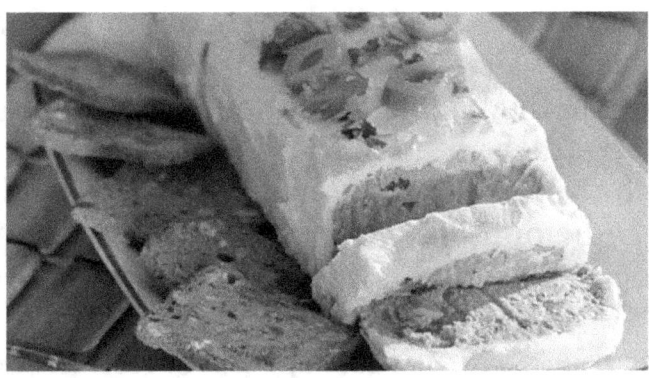

8 servings

Nutrients per 100 g:

- Total Carbohydrates – 3 g
- Fat – 35.5 g
- Protein – 11.2 g
- Calories – 373.3

Ingredients:

- 1 package softened cream cheese
- 1 tablespoon chopped green onion
- 2 tablespoons softened butter
- 1/4 teaspoon Worcestershire sauce
- 2 slices bacon, cooked and crumbled
- 8 oz. liverwurst sausage

Directions:

1. Preheat the oven to 375 °F. Cook the bacon strips on a baking tray for 15 minutes. Transfer from the oven and set aside to cool down. Reserve the grease.

2. Crumble the bacon very finely.

3. Stir together green onion, Worcestershire sauce, butter, bacon, and liverwurst in a medium bowl. Ladle onto waxed paper. Shape into a 3x5 inch rectangle. Freeze the mixture for 30 minutes to set.

4. Over the top and sides, spread softened cheese cream. Refrigerate for 30 minutes then serve.

Stilton and Chive Pate

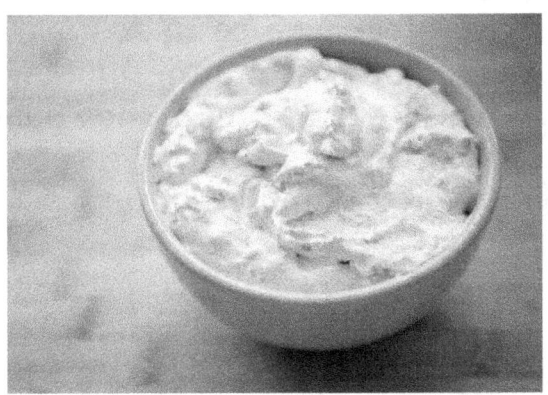

6 servings

Nutrients per 100 g:

- Total Carbohydrates – 2.1 g
- Fat – 39 g
- Protein – 8.6 g
- Calories – 387.4

Ingredients:

- 3.5 oz. full-fat cream cheese, at room temperature
- 2 oz. unsalted butter, at room temperature
- 2.3 oz. crumbled Stilton or other blue cheese
- 1.1 oz. chopped fresh chives
- 1 tablespoon chopped fresh parsley

Directions:
1. Combine the cream cheese and butter, or process in a food processor until smooth.
2. Add the cheese, spring onions, and parsley.
3. Mix until well combined.
4. Refrigerate for 30 minutes, or until set. Serve and enjoy.

Bacon & Egg Pate

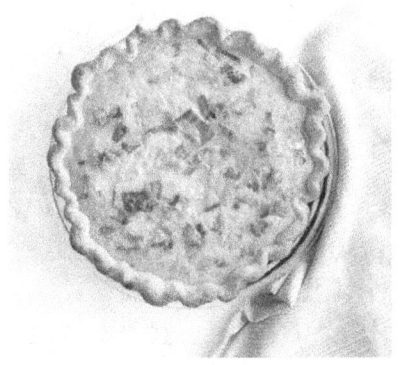

5 servings

Nutrients per 100 g:
- Total Carbohydrates – 1 g
- Fat – 46.3 g
- Protein – 20.7 g
- Calories – 487.6

Ingredients:
- 2 large eggs
- 1/4 cup butter, softened
- 2 tablespoons mayonnaise
- freshly ground black pepper, optional
- 1/4 teaspoon salt or to taste
- 4 large slices bacon

Directions:

1. Boil the eggs in salt water for 10 minutes. Remove from the heat and place them in a bowl with cold water. Chill and peel off the shells.
2. Cook the bacon slices until crispy. Transfer the slices to a plate and leave them to cool. Reserve the grease.
3. Crumble the bacon very finely.
4. Crush the eggs with a fork in a bowl.
5. Add the mayonnaise, bacon, salt, bacon grease, and pepper. Combine well.
6. Cover and place to the fridge for 20 minutes or so before serving.

Desserts

From time to time, you can treat yourself to your favorite desserts even while keeping a Keto diet. This book presents some of the most popular desserts.

Chocolate Chip Cookies

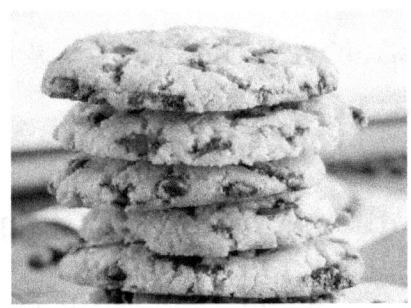

6 servings

Nutrients per serving:
- Total Carbohydrates – 2.3 g
- Fat – 17.3 g
- Protein – 4 g
- Calories – 168

Ingredients:
- 6 oz. almond meal
- 3.5 oz. salted butter
- 4.5 oz. erythritol
- 1 teaspoon vanilla extract
- 1 large egg

- 1/2 teaspoon baking powder
- 1/4 teaspoon salt
- 1/2 teaspoon xanthan gum (optional)
- 3 oz. sugar free chocolate chips

Directions:

1. Preheat your oven to 355 F.
2. Melt the butter for 30 seconds, but it shouldn't be hot.
3. Beat the butter with the erythritol in a mixing bowl.
4. Add the vanilla and egg, beat in well on low speed.
5. Add the xanthan gum, almond flour, baking powder, and salt and mix until well combined.
6. Combine the chocolate chips into the dough.
7. Make 12 balls (with your hands or an ice cream scoop) and place on a baking tray lined with a parchment paper. Bake for 10 minutes (your cookies melt in the oven).
8. Let them cool, and serve.

Peach Cobbler

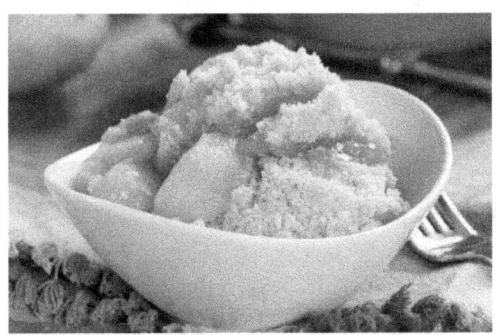

6 servings

Nutrients per serving:
- Total Carbohydrates – 12 g
- Fat – 25 g
- Protein – 7 g
- Calories – 275

Ingredients:
- 3 fresh ripe peaches, sliced (peeled, if desired)
- 2 tsp tapioca starch optional
- Sprinkle of cinnamon
- Sprinkle of pure stevia powder

Topping:
- 1 1/2 cups almond flour
- 1/4 cup coconut oil
- 2 tablespoons coconut milk

- 1/8 teaspoon pure stevia powder
- 1 tablespoon ground flaxseed
- 2 tablespoons water
- Pinch of salt

Directions:
1. Preheat oven to 375 F.
2. Grease 8x6 glass baking dish. Peel and slice the peaches in the dish, sprinkle with starch, cinnamon, and stevia and stir to coat. Set aside.
3. Mix water and flax in a small bowl. Set aside to thicken.
4. Stir together almond flour, stevia, and salt in a medium mixing bowl.
5. Then pour on coconut milk, oil, and flax mixture. Mix well.
6. Place topping over peaches and smooth with a spatula.
7. Bake for 20-25 minutes. The topping should be lightly golden.
8. Allow to cool, serve and enjoy.

Vanilla Ice Cream

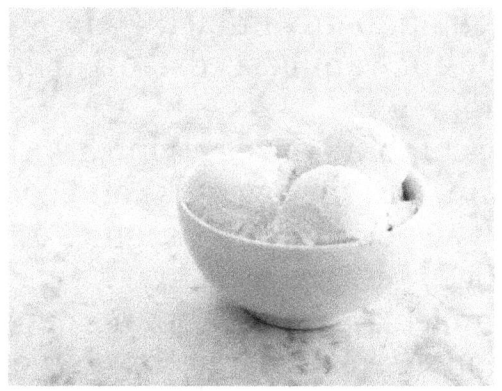

6 servings

Nutrients per serving:
- Total Carbohydrates – 5 g
- Fat – 12 g
- Protein – 5 g
- Calories – 137

Ingredients:
- 4 eggs separated
- 1 1/3 cup heavy cream
- 1/3 cup erythritol
- 1 vanilla bean

Directions:
1. Separate the whites from the yolks.
2. Beat egg whites into a thick foam.
3. Mix the erythritol with the egg whites.

4. Whip the heavy cream in a separate bowl. When the cream becomes thicker than usual (but not butter), stop to mix immediately.

5. Scrape out the vanilla seeds. Mix them with the heavy cream.

6. Carefully combine the egg whites with the beaten cream, and the egg yolks and continue mixing with a spoon until it becomes a homogeneous mass.

7. Place in an ice cream tray or another suitable rectangle pan. Freeze for 4 hours. Serve and enjoy!

Strawberry Cheesecake

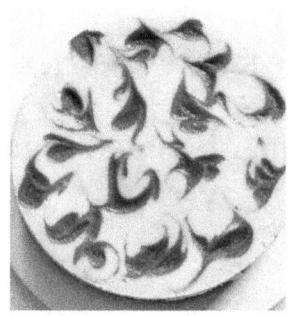

8 servings
Nutrients per serving:
- Net Carbohydrates – 3 g
- Fat – 23 g
- Protein – 4 g
- Calories – 239

Ingredients:
For the crust:
- 6 tablespoons butter, softened
- 1/2 cup granulated sugar substitute (Swerve)
- 1/2 cup desiccated unsweetened coconut
- 1/4 cup coconut flour
- 1/2 teaspoon baking powder

For the filling:
- 8 oz. cream cheese
- 1/3 cup granulated sugar substitute (Swerve)

- 1 tablespoon lemon juice
- 1 egg

For the strawberry swirl:
- 1/2 cup pureed strawberries (about 3/4 cup chopped)
- 1 tablespoon granulated sugar substitute (Swerve)

Directions:
1. Mix the butter and the sweetener.
2. Add the coconut flour, coconut, and baking powder. Mix until thoroughly combined.
3. Grease nonstick springform pan (8 inches or slightly smaller). Press the mixture into the springform forming the crust. Set aside.
4. Preheat the oven to 350 F.
5. Whip the cream cheese and the sweetener until smooth.
6. Add lemon juice and the egg and mix until thoroughly combined.
7. Pour the cheesecake filling over the crust.
8. Combine the strawberry puree and one tablespoon of sweetener.
9. Drop the strawberry puree by spoonful over the filling and then swirl gently with a knife or fork. Don't over mix.
10. Bake for 30 minutes. Serve and enjoy!

Easy Chocolate Cheesecake

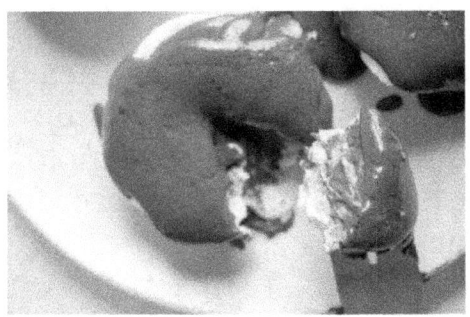

4 servings

Nutrients per serving:

- Total Carbohydrates – 5.2 g
- Fat – 29 g
- Protein – 4.2 g
- Calories – 323

Ingredients:

For the filling:

- 4 oz. 1/3 less fat Philadelphia Cream Cheese
- 2 tablespoons sour cream
- 1/4 cup heavy whipping cream
- 1/4 cup erythritol

For the ganache:

- 2 oz. unsweetened baker's chocolate
- 1/2 cup heavy whipping cream

- splash of water

Directions:
1. Mix cream cheese, sour cream, heavy whipping cream, and erythritol with a hand mixer.
2. Spoon the filling into cupcake molds and place in the fridge for 2-3 hours or freezer for 1-2 hours. For the ganache:
3. Melt baker's chocolate in a microwave.
4. Add heavy whipping cream, a splash of water and combine well until you get a thick liquid consistency.
5. Pour over top frozen cheesecakes and serve.

Strawberry Cream Pie

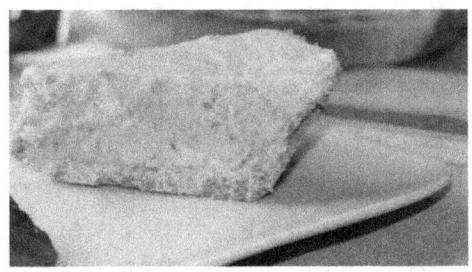

10 servings
Nutrients per serving:
- Total Carbohydrates – 6.2 g
- Fat – 21.1 g
- Protein – 4.8 g
- Calories – 233

Ingredients:
For the crust:
- 1 1/2 cups almond flour
- 1/4 cup powdered Swerve Sweetener
- 1/4 teaspoon salt
- 1/4 cup butter, melted

For the strawberry cream filling:
- 1 1/2 cups fresh strawberries, chopped
- 1/4 cup water
- 2 1/2 teaspoons grass-fed gelatin
- 1 cup heavy whipping cream
- 1/2 cup powdered Swerve Sweetener
- 3/4 teaspoon vanilla extract

Directions:

For the crust:

1. Mix almond flour, sweetener, and salt in a medium bowl.
2. Pour on melted butter and mix until the dough comes together and looks like coarse crumbs.
3. Scrape the crust mixture into a pie plate. Form the crust with fingers into the bottom and up sides. Smooth out the bottom using a flat-bottomed glass or measuring cup.
4. Place to the fridge and freeze while making the filling.

For the strawberry cream filling:

5. Process the strawberries with the water in a blender or a food processor.
6. Transfer the puree to a medium saucepan and beat in the gelatin with a whisk.
7. Heat over low heat, whisking to dissolve the gelatin. Don't boil the puree!
8. Cool for 20 minutes.
9. Mix the cream, sweetener, and vanilla extract. Beat into a thick foam.
10. Pour in the strawberry mixture and blend until well combined.
11. Spoon into the prepared crust and refrigerate about 3 hours until firm.
12. Serve with fresh berries.

Indiana Sugar Cream Pie

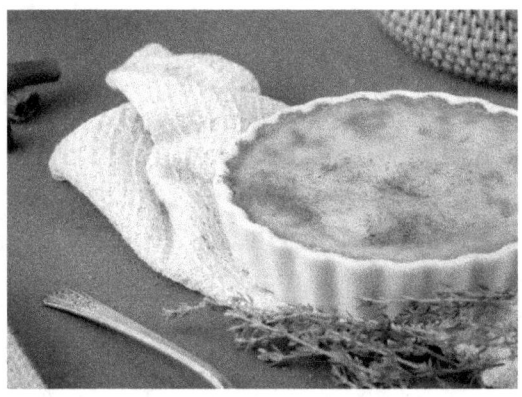

8 servings
Nutrients per serving:
- Total Carbohydrates – 2 g
- Fat – 18 g
- Protein – 3 g
- Calories – 200

Ingredients:
For the crust:
- 1 1/4 cups almond flour
- 4 tablespoons butter, melted
- 2 tablespoons Lakanto Golden Monkfruit Sweetener

For the filling:
- 2 cups heavy cream
- 3/4 cups Lakanto Golden Monkfruit Sweetener

- 1 teaspoon organic vanilla extract
- 1 teaspoon salt

Directions:
1. Preheat oven to 400°F.
2. Mix almond flour, melted butter, the sweetener in a bowl.
3. Form a crust in a pie plate.
4. Bake the crust for 8 minutes.
5. Combine heavy cream, sweetener, vanilla extract, and salt into a pot and heat it over low heat. Stir the filling occasionally and don't boil it. The sweetener must be completely dissolved.
6. Pour the filling mixture over the crust.
7. Bake for 50-60 minutes, until the cream has turned a light golden color.
8. Remove the pie from the oven, let it cool and chill it at least 4 hours before serving.

Mocha Cheesecake Bars

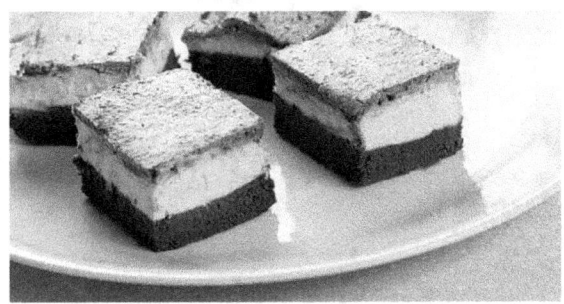

16 servings
Nutrients per serving:
- Net Carbohydrates – 3.2 g
- Fat – 21 g
- Protein – 6.1 g
- Calories – 232

Ingredients:
For the brownie layer:
- 6 tablespoons unsalted butter
- 2 teaspoons vanilla extract
- 3 large eggs
- 1 cup erythritol
- 1 1/2 cups almond flour
- 1/2 tablespoon instant coffee
- 1/2 cup Hershey's Baking Cocoa
- 1/2 teaspoon salt
- 1 teaspoon baking powder

For the cream cheese layer:
- 1 pound cream cheese, softened
- 1/2 cup erythritol
- 1 teaspoon vanilla extract
- 1 large egg

Directions:
1. Preheat oven to 350°F.
2. Spray or grease an 8×8-inch baking pan.
3. In a mixing bowl, mix the melted unsalted butter and two teaspoons of vanilla extract until well combined. Then mix in the three large eggs.
4. In a small bowl, mix almond flour, instant coffee, baking cocoa, salt, erythritol, and baking powder.
5. Combine two mixtures and whisk thoroughly. Reserve 1/4 cup of batter to use later.
6. Add the larger portion of batter into the 8x8-inch baking pan.
7. Combine the cream cheese, one large egg, one teaspoon vanilla extract, and 1/2 cup erythritol in a mixing bowl. Mix until well incorporated.
8. Spread on top of the brownie layer.
9. Mix the 1/4 cup of brownie batter into the top layer of cream cheese to create a top brownie crust. This layer should be very thin.
10. Bake for 30-35 minutes at 350°F.
11. Cool the cheesecake and then slice it. Serve and enjoy!

Brownies

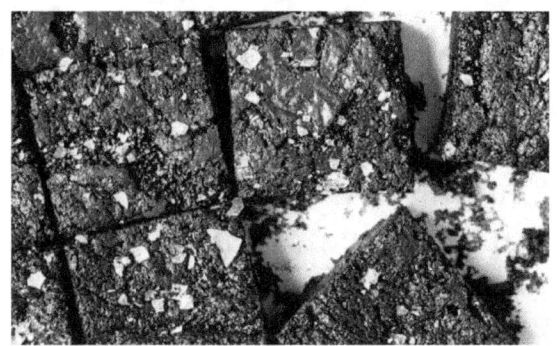

16 servings
Nutrients per serving:
- Total Carbohydrates – 3 g
- Fat – 9 g
- Protein – 2 g
- Calories – 102

Ingredients:
- 130 g unsalted grass-fed butter or 8 tablespoons coconut oil
- 140-200 g xylitol
- 80 g cocoa powder
- 1/2 teaspoon salt
- 2 eggs at room temperature
- 70 g almond flour

Directions:
1. Preheat your oven to 350°F.

2. Melt over a water bath butter, sweetener, cocoa powder, and salt whisking constantly. Heat the mixture until most of the sweetener has melted.

3. Remove from heat and cool the mixture.

4. Add an egg at a time. Whisk well after each one until completely incorporated. All the sweetener must dissolve into the mixture.

5. Add the almond flour, blend until well incorporated.

6. Cover with parchment paper an 8x8-inch baking pan (the bottom and sides). Pour on the mixture into the pan.

7. Bake for 15-25 minutes. Check out for the first time on the 15th minute of baking. If a toothpick inserted in the center comes out clean, the brownies are cooked.

8. Place brownies on an oven rack. Let the brownies to cool completely.

9. Freeze for 10 minutes before cutting into slices.

Chocolate Chunk Cookies

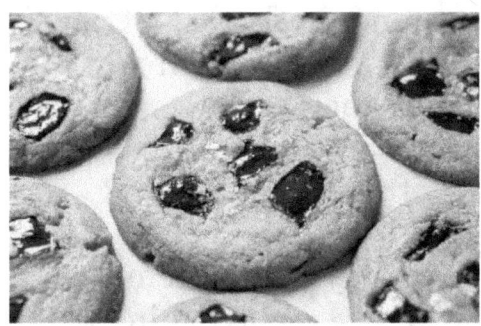

11 servings

Nutrients per serving:
- Total Carbohydrates – 3.75 g
- Fat – 16 g
- Protein – 6 g
- Calories – 183

Ingredients:
- 57 g grass-fed butter at room temperature
- 1/2 cup Swerve or xylitol
- 1 teaspoon vanilla extract
- 1/2 teaspoon baking soda
- 1/2 teaspoon kosher salt
- 1 egg
- 320 g shelled and roasted peanuts
- chocolate chunks or chips to taste

Directions:

1. Process peanuts until smooth in the food processor.
2. Cream sweetener and 270 g of peanut butter in a large bowl with an electric mixer.
3. Add vanilla extract, baking soda, egg, and salt and mix well.
4. Cover and refrigerate for 1 hour.
5. Preheat oven to 350°F.
6. Line a baking tray with parchment paper.
7. Spoon the dough on the baking tray.
8. Add in chocolate chunks and level out with a spoon.
9. Place the cookies into freezer for 15 minutes before baking.
10. Bake for 8-10 minutes, but only until they just begin to brown around the edges. Not let them brown!
11. Let them cool completely and serve.

Peanut Butter Balls

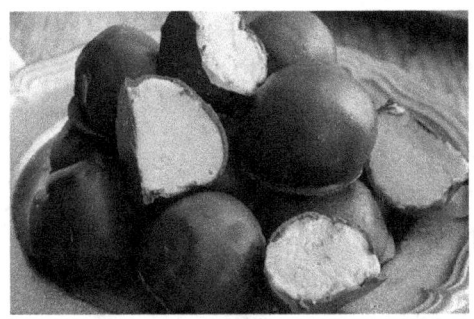

15 servings
Nutrients per serving:
- Total Carbohydrates – 6.9 g
- Fat – 15.1 g
- Protein – 7.2 g
- Calories – 180

Ingredients:
- 1 cup peanut butter
- 1 cup almond flour
- 1/4 cup powdered erythritol/swerve confectioners
- 3 oz. unsweetened bakers' chocolate

Directions:

1. Mix well peanut butter, almond flour, and sweetener.
2. Freeze peanut butter mixture for an hour.
3. Melt baker's chocolate in the microwave.
4. Roll frozen peanut butter mixture into balls. If peanut butter balls seem too soft, return it to the refrigerator for 20-30 minutes.
5. Cover the dish with wax paper. Dip the balls into melted chocolate one by one and place on the dish.
6. Refrigerate the balls until they harden. Serve and enjoy!

Pancakes

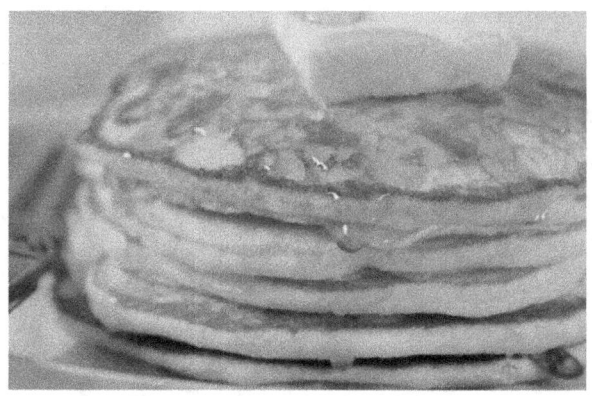

10 servings

Nutrients per serving:

- Total Carbohydrates – 2 g
- Fat – 10 g
- Protein – 4 g
- Calories – 118

Ingredients:

- 1 cup almond flour
- 4 large whole eggs
- 1/4 cup unsweetened almond milk
- 1 teaspoon pure vanilla extract
- 1/2 teaspoon baking powder
- 2 tablespoons oil

Directions:

1. Mix almond flour, eggs, almond milk, vanilla extract, baking powder with a whisk or hand mixer.
2. Heat the oil in a large skillet. Pour on 1/4 cup of pancake mixture onto the skillet and brown a pancake on both sides.
3. Serve hot with berries or syrups that are allowed in the Keto diet.

Cupcakes

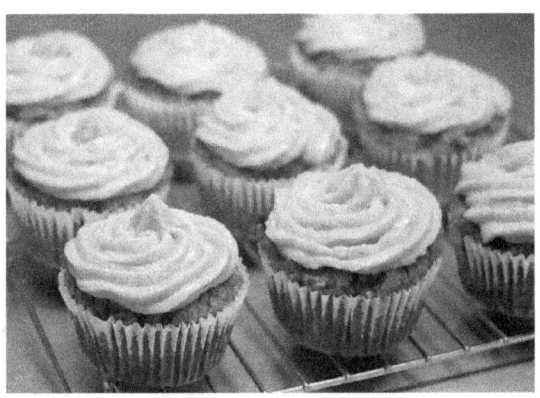

18 servings

Nutrients per serving:
- Total Carbohydrates – 3 g
- Fat – 16 g
- Protein – 2 g
- Calories – 160

Ingredients:

For the cupcakes:
- 2/3 cup almond meal
- 3 tablespoons cocoa powder unsweetened
- 1 1/2 tablespoons baking powder
- 3 tablespoons natvia
- 1 tablespoon sugar free maple syrup
- 2 oz. heavy cream
- 2 eggs

- 2 oz. butter unsalted, melted

For the frosting:
- 5 oz. butter unsalted, softened
- 3 oz. natvia icing mix
- 2 tablespoons heavy cream

Directions:

For the cupcakes:

1. Preheat fan forced oven to 350F.
2. Mix almond meal, cocoa powder, baking powder, and natvia with a hand mixer on low speed until combined.
3. Combine maple syrup, heavy cream, eggs, and melted butter in a bowl.
4. Add almond meal, cocoa powder, baking powder, natvia to the bowl with the wet ingredients and mix until well combined.
5. Line a mini muffin tray with the liners and spoon dough into the papers until they are 3/4 full.
6. Bake in the oven for 10 to 14 minutes, until a toothpick inserted into the center of a cupcake, comes out clean.
7. Cool the cupcakes.

For the frosting:

8. Let your butter to soften at room temperature. Cut the softened butter into cubes and place into a bowl.

9. Beat the butter with a mixer for 3 minutes on low speed, just until it's smooth.

10. Add the natvia icing mix (one spoon at a time, so you don't end up throwing it all over the place), until all the icing mix has been included into the butter.

11. Add the heavy cream and mix the frosting for 3 minutes. Scrape sides and bottom of bowl often to ensure the frosting is thoroughly mixed.

12. Decorate the cooled cupcakes.

Chocolate Chip Muffins

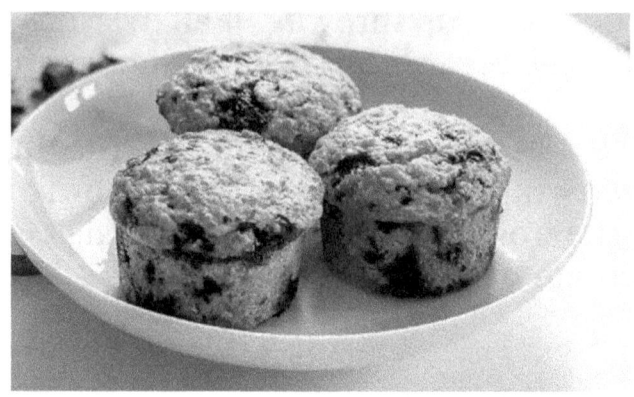

12 servings

Nutrients per serving:
- Total Carbohydrates – 6 g
- Fat – 25 g
- Protein – 8 g
- Calories – 277

Ingredients:
- 3 cups almond flour (360 g)
- 1 teaspoon baking soda
- 1 1/2 teaspoons baking powder
- 1/2 cup ghee, melted
- 4 eggs
- 1/4 cup erythritol
- 1 cup 100% dark chocolate, chopped into very small cubes (85 g)

- 1 tablespoon vanilla extract (15 ml)

Directions:
1. Preheat oven to 350 F.
2. Whip the eggs.
3. Add the almond flour, baking soda, baking powder, ghee, erythritol, and vanilla extract to the eggs. Mix well.
4. Fold in the chocolate cubes.
5. Use a muffin pan with muffin liners, silicone muffin liners or grease well a muffin pan.
6. Spoon the mixture into the forms for three quarters and level out with a spoon.
7. Bake for 15 minutes. Check the muffin with a toothpick (it must come out clean inserted in the center). Serve and enjoy!

Chocolate Peanut Butter Pecan Bark

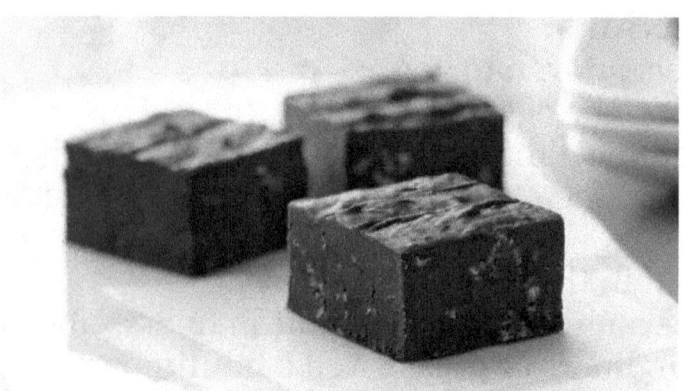

25 servings
Nutrients per serving:
- Total Carbohydrates – 6 g (with pecans - 7 g)
- Fat – 12 g (with pecans – 14.2 g)
- Protein – 1.5 g (with pecans – 1.8 g)
- Calories – 116 (with pecans – 135)

Ingredients:
- 1 cup coconut oil
- 1/4 cup unsweetened cocoa powder
- 1/2 cup creamy peanut butter (sugar free)
- 1/2 cup Swerve (or stevia)
- 1/4 teaspoon sea salt
- 1 teaspoon vanilla extract
- 1 teaspoon almond extract
- 1/2 cups shredded coconut unsweetened

- 1/2 cup pecans (optional)

Directions:
1. Melt peanut butter and the coconut oil until creamy, and no chunks of coconut oil remain. Stir well.
2. Add the sea salt, sweetener, shredded coconut, almond extract, vanilla extract, and cocoa powder. Mix well.
3. Pour the melted chocolate on a baking tray lined with a parchment paper. Gently press the pecan into the chocolate (optional).
4. Freeze the chocolate for 45 minutes.
5. Break into pieces. Store the desert in the freezer.

Conclusion

I want to thank you for buying my book.
I hope that the dishes from the book
diversify your Keto diet and allow you
to indulge yourself with your favorite dishes.

www.ingramcontent.com/pod-product-compliance
Lightning Source LLC
Chambersburg PA
CBHW051312220526
45468CB00004B/1313